Facial Gender Affirmation Surgery

Editor

MICHAEL T. SOMENEK

FACIAL PLASTIC SURGERY CLINICS OF NORTH AMERICA

www.facialplastic.theclinics.com

Consulting Editor
J. REGAN THOMAS

May 2019 • Volume 27 • Number 2

ELSEVIER

1600 John F. Kennedy Boulevard ● Suite 1800 ● Philadelphia, Pennsylvania, 19103-2899

http://www.theclinics.com

FACIAL PLASTIC SURGERY CLINICS OF NORTH AMERICA Volume 27, Number 2
May 2019 ISSN 1064-7406, ISBN-13: 978-0-323-65521-7

Editor: Jessica McCool
Developmental Editor: Sara Watkins

Facial Plastic Surgery Clinics of North America (ISSN 1064-7406) is published quarterly by Elsevier Inc., 360 Park Avenue South, New York, NY 10010-1710. Months of issue are February, May, August, and November. Business and Editorial Offices: 1600 John F. Kennedy Blvd., Suite 1800, Philadelphia, PA 19103-2899. Periodicals postage paid at New York, NY, and additional mailing offices. Subscription prices are $408.00 per year (US individuals), $659.00 per year (US institutions), $454.00 per year (Canadian individuals), $820.00 per year (Canadian institutions), $535.00 per year (foreign individuals), $820.00 per year (foreign institutions), $100.00 per year (US students), and $255.00 per year (foreign students). Foreign air speed delivery is included in all *Clinics* subscription prices. All prices are subject to change without notice. POSTMASTER: Send address changes to *Facial Plastic Surgery Clinics*, Elsevier Health Sciences Division, Subscription Customer Service, 3251 Riverport Lane, Maryland Heights, MO 63043. **Customer service: 1-800-654-2452 (US and Canada); 1-314-447-8871 (outside US and Canada); Fax: 314-447-8029; E-mail: journalscustomerservice-usa@elsevier.com (for print support); journalsonline support-usa@elsevier.com (for online support).**

Reprints. For copies of 100 or more of articles in this publication, please contact the Commercial Reprints Department, Elsevier Inc., 360 Park Avenue South, New York, NY 10010-1710. Tel.: 212-633-3874; Fax: 212-633-3820; E-mail: reprints@elsevier.com.

Facial Plastic Surgery Clinics of North America is covered in *MEDLINE/PubMed* (*Index Medicus*).

Contributors

CONSULTING EDITOR

J. REGAN THOMAS, MD
Professor, Facial Plastic and Reconstructive
Surgery, Department of Otolaryngology–Head
and Neck Surgery, Northwestern University
Feinberg School of Medicine, Chicago, Illinois,
USA

EDITOR

MICHAEL T. SOMENEK, MD
SomenekMD-Advanced Facial Plastic Surgery,
Washington, DC, USA

AUTHORS

ANTHONY BARED, MD, FACS
Private Practice, Foundation for Hair
Restoration, Miami, Florida, USA

JENS URS BERLI, MD
Division of Plastic and Reconstructive Surgery,
Department of General Surgery, Oregon Health
& Science University, Portland, Oregon, USA

RACHEL BLUEBOND-LANGNER, MD
Hansjörg Wyss Department of Plastic Surgery,
New York University Langone Health, New
York, New York, USA

SCOTT R. CHAIET, MD, MBA
Assistant Professor, Division of
Otolaryngology–Head and Neck Surgery,
Department of Surgery, University of
Wisconsin-Madison School of Medicine and
Public Health, Madison, Wisconsin, USA

JORDAN DESCHAMPS-BRALY, MD, FACS
Deschamps-Braly Clinic of Plastic &
Craniofacial Surgery, San Francisco,
California, USA

MARCELO DI MAGGIO, MD
Director, MDM Surgery Center, Sanatorio
Finochietto Medical Center, Buenos Aires,
Argentina

JAMES M. ECONOMIDES, MD
Department of Plastic and Reconstructive
Surgery, MedStar Georgetown University
Hospital, Pasquerilla Health Center,
Washington, DC, USA

JEFFREY S. EPSTEIN, MD, FACS
Private Practice, Foundation for
Hair Restoration, Miami, Florida,
USA

RONNI HAYON, MD
Assistant Professor, Department of Family
Medicine and Community Health, University
of Wisconsin-Madison, Madison, Wisconsin,
USA

MAARTEN J. KOUDSTAAL, MD, DMD, PhD
Department of Craniofacial Diseases,
Karolinska University Hospital, Department
for Molecular Medicine and Surgery,
Karolinska Institutet, Stockholm,
Sweden

CHRISOVALANTIS LAKHIANI, MD
MedStar Georgetown University Hospital,
Washington, DC, USA

MYRIAM LOYO, MD
Assistant Professor, Division of Facial Plastic and Reconstructive Surgery, Department of Otolaryngology–Head and Neck Surgery, Oregon Health & Science University, Portland, Oregon, USA

KALLE CONNERYD LUNDGREN, MD, PhD
Department of Craniofacial Diseases, Karolinska University Hospital, Department for Molecular Medicine and Surgery, Karolinska Institutet, Stockholm, Sweden

SHANE D. MORRISON, MD, MS
Resident Physician, Division of Plastic Surgery, Department of Surgery, University of Washington School of Medicine, Seattle, Washington, USA

TROY A. PITTMAN, MD
Advanced Plastic Surgery, Washington, DC, USA

ARA A. SALIBIAN, MD
Hansjörg Wyss Department of Plastic Surgery, New York University Langone Health, New York, New York, USA

THOMAS SATTERWHITE, MD
Surgeon, Brownstein and Crane Surgical Services, San Francisco, California, USA

LOREN S. SCHECHTER, MD, FACS
Clinical Professor of Surgery, The University of Illinois at Chicago, Director, The Center for Gender Confirmation Surgery, Weiss Memorial Hospital, Morton Grove, Illinois, USA

MICHAEL T. SOMENEK, MD
SomenekMD-Advanced Facial Plastic Surgery, Washington, DC, USA

KRISTIN STEVENSON, MD
Fellow, Department of Medicine, Division of Endocrinology, Diabetes & Metabolism, University of Wisconsin-Madison, Madison, Wisconsin, USA

ANGELA STURM, MD
Assistant Professor, Department of Otolaryngology–Head and Neck Surgery, University of Texas Medical Branch, Galveston, Texas, USA; Private Practice, Facial Plastic Surgery Associates, Houston, Texas, USA

DAVID M. WHITEHEAD, MD, MS
Assistant Professor, Division of Plastic Surgery, Department of Surgery, Donald and Barbara Zucker School of Medicine at Hofstra/Northwell, North New Hyde Park, New York, USA

Contents

Foreword: Facial Gender Affirmation Surgery   ix

J. Regan Thomas

Preface: Exploring Facial Gender Affirmation Surgery   xi

Michael T. Somenek

Gender-related Facial Analysis   171

Chrisovalantis Lakhiani and Michael T. Somenek

> There exist several known anthropometric differences between the male and female facial skeleton and soft tissues. In general, the female face is less robust, rounder or heart shaped, with a shorter forehead, no supraorbital bossing, a smaller nose, more pronounced zygomatic prominences, fuller lips, a smaller mandibular width, and a more tapered chin. A method for analyzing these differences is critical for offering facial gender confirming surgery to the gender dysphoric patients, both for preoperative planning, as well as for setting postoperative expectations.

Hormonal, Medical, and Nonsurgical Aspects of Gender Affirmation   179

Ronni Hayon and Kristin Stevenson

> Although the acronym LGBTQ is often used as a catchall label for sexual and gender minorities, transgender people have unique and individual health needs and, unfortunately, experience significant health disparities. This article reviews essential terminology and concepts relevant to discussions of gender and gender identity, practical tips for changes that can be made on both clinical and institutional levels in order to create a welcoming and safe environment for transgender patients, as well as current recommendations for the provision of gender-affirming medical therapy.

Preparing for Facial Feminization Surgery: Timing   191

Troy A. Pittman and James M. Economides

> Facial feminization surgery may be a part of a treatment plan for gender dysphoria. Initial mental health assessment must occur. Referrals for hormonal therapy may then be made if appropriate. No guidelines exist for timing of facial feminization surgery. Generally, recommendations are for individuals to undergo hormonal therapy and live in a gender-congruent role for at least 12 months before surgical intervention. Referral letters meeting World Professional Association of Transgender Health guidelines must be made regarding the treatment course and goals. Informed consent must be obtained; patient should understand how surgical alteration fits into their overall treatment goals.

Cheek Augmentation Techniques   199

David M. Whitehead and Loren S. Schechter

> The restoration of a youthful appearance to the midface can enhance its femininity. In this article, we discuss several strategies and techniques, both surgical and nonsurgical, for augmentation of the lateral and centro-lateral midface.

Forehead and Orbital Rim Remodeling   207

Marcelo Di Maggio

> Facial features remodeling surgery is performed to obtain feminization of the face
> that corresponds to the gender perceived by patients. This includes techniques
> and findings to remodel the forehead and orbital rim to change the expression of
> the eyes, correction of the frontonasal angle in relation to rhinoplasty, hairline femi-
> nization, and eyebrow lift to correct the position and aesthetic dissatisfaction or the
> effects of aging.

Midfacial Bony Remodeling   221

Kalle Conneryd Lundgren and Maarten J. Koudstaal

> Craniofacial procedures to the midface in conjunction with work to the upper face
> and skull, and if needed the lower jaw, are a permanent and effective way to achieve
> feminization of the face in transgender patients. Although the surgery is more com-
> plex than other procedures, it should be considered for select patients. Further
> improvement of cosmesis may be considered a separate surgical entity and is not
> limited in scope or time by having undergone midface osteotomies. When carefully
> planned, bony surgery to the midface is safe and results in long-term predictive re-
> sults and a favorable appearance as the patient ages.

Hair Transplantation Techniques for the Transgender Patient   227

Anthony Bared and Jeffrey S. Epstein

> Hair transplantation can play a complementary role in the spectrum of gender trans-
> formation procedures sought by transgender patients undergoing gender transfor-
> mation surgery. The authors' clinic has seen an increase in the demand for hair
> restoration in transgender patients. Hairline lowering, eyebrow transplantation,
> and pubic hair transplantation can play roles for male-to-female transgender pa-
> tients whereas beard hair transplantation and body hair transplantation can play in-
> tegral roles for female-to-male patients seeking gender transformation surgery. This
> article delineates an experience in the role hair restoration plays for transgender pa-
> tients and outlines a surgical approach for these hair restoration procedures.

Lower Jaw Recontouring in Facial Gender-Affirming Surgery   233

Shane D. Morrison and Thomas Satterwhite

> Facial gender-affirming surgery can have significant impact on patient quality of life
> for some gender-dysphoric patients. Lower jaw contouring can be used to harmo-
> nize the face during facial gender-affirming surgery through masculinization or femi-
> nization. During feminization, the mandibular angle and body and chin are reduced in
> width and size. During masculinization, augmentation of the mandibular angle and
> body and chin are completed with alloplastic implants, fat, or bone. Complications
> are minimal. Further research is needed on outcomes of these procedures.

Feminization of the Chin: Genioplasty Using Osteotomies   243

Jordan Deschamps-Braly

> Chin reshaping can provide a more identifiable female appearance for transitioning
> male to female patients undergoing facial feminization. The "sliding" genioplasty has
> the most potential for dramatically reshaping the chin, while also avoiding many of

the issues that may occur with implants. A chin should be evaluated radiologically and by physical examination to determine what changes should be made to any particular chin. When performing osseous genioplasty, the mental nerve can be protected by performing any osteotomies at least 6 mm below the inferior border of the mental nerve canal.

Gender confirming Rhinoplasty

251

Jens Urs Berli and Myriam Loyo

Most surgeons who are not routinely treating gender dysphoric patients are more likely to see an isolated rhinoplasty consultation rather than a request for full facial gender confirmation surgery (FGCS). Different from other aspects of FGCS, the surgical basis of rhinoplasty is almost the same as for the cisgender population. Despite technical overlap, the care for patients seeking rhinoplasty for the indication of gender dysphoria vastly differs from that for the cisgender population. This review includes comments on gender norms and outline considerations for the preoperative work-up and operative execution as well as a comprehensive literature review.

Lip Lift

261

Ara A. Salibian and Rachel Bluebond-Langner

The male upper lip has a distinctly longer cutaneous height from the nasal base to the upper vermilion border than its female counterpart. The subnasal indirect lip lift using the bullhorn technique or its modifications allows for shortening of this height to feminize the lower face, creating a more aesthetically pleasing upper lip secondary to increased vermilion height and lip pout. Patient selection is critical, taking into account lip height, vermilion height, alar base width, skin type, upper incisal show, and maxillary height. Precise measurements, controlled excision of the planned resection, and meticulous reapproximation of skin provide an aesthetic result, while minimizing visible scarring.

Chondrolaryngoplasty—Thyroid Cartilage Reduction

267

Angela Sturm and Scott R. Chaiet

Chondrolaryngoplasty, also known as tracheal shave, is a surgical procedure performed for a prominent Adam's apple, usually in transfeminine patients with gender dysphoria to this marker of male sex. Although laryngeal anatomy is complex, knowledge of landmarks and techniques discussed in this article results in a safe procedure with rare complications and improvement in quality of life.

FACIAL PLASTIC SURGERY CLINICS OF NORTH AMERICA

FORTHCOMING ISSUES

August 2019
**New Trends and Technologies in Facial
Plastic Surgery**
Jason D. Bloom, *Editor*

November 2019
**Revision Facial Plastic Surgery: Correcting
Bad Results**
Paul S. Nassif and Julia L. Kerolus, *Editors*

February 2020
**Update of Todays Facial Skin Rejuvenation
Technology**
Richard Gentile, *Editor*

RECENT ISSUES

February 2019
Skin Cancer Treatment
Jeffrey S. Moyer, *Editor*

November 2018
Current Utilization of Biologicals
Gregory S. Keller, *Editor*

August 2018
Rhinoplasty for the Asian Nose
Yong Ju Jang, *Editor*

Foreword
Facial Gender Affirmation Surgery

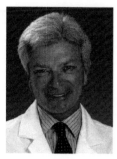

J. Regan Thomas, MD
Consulting Editor

A key component for those individuals who have elected to undergo procedures to address gender dysmorphia is facial modification surgery. Gender dysphoria may cause people to experience major stress and impairment on social and personal levels. For these individuals, gender role changing, including surgery, may permit their outside appearance to match what they feel internally. Gender dysmorphia, previously referred to as gender identity disorder, often is assisted through the skills and procedures provided by facial plastic surgery. Individuals with gender dysphoria often describe themselves as being born in the wrong body and hope that plastic surgery will align their appearance with whom they know themselves to be.

In this issue of *Facial Plastic Surgery Clinics of North America*, guest editor Dr Michael Somenek and the participating authors review techniques and treatments that may assist this population adapt and deal with their personal transformation of gender identification. This group of individuals with gender dysmorphia is increasingly being recognized, and it is hoped that surgeons providing transgender care are able to enhance an improved quality of life and positive self-identification by gender dysmorphic patients. The overall goal of this issue is to not only describe treatment modalities utilized in assisting these individuals but also help physicians understand the importance of supporting gender dysmorphic patients in their pursuit of an improved quality of life through positive self-identification and interaction with others in the world around them.

Dr Somenek and the contributing authors have actively organized and described a sophisticated and updated approach to serving this group of individuals from a variety of perspectives and enhanced treatment modality utilization. I hope you find this issue of *Facial Plastic Surgery Clinics of North America* informative, insightful, and beneficial in your approach to serving these patients.

J. Regan Thomas, MD
Facial Plastic and Reconstructive Surgery
Department of Otolaryngology
Head and Neck Surgery
Northwestern University School of Medicine
675 North Saint Clair Street
Suite 15-200
Chicago, IL 60611, USA

E-mail address:
regan.thomas@nm.org

https://doi.org/10.1016/j.fsc.2019.02.002

facialplastic.theclinics.com

Preface
Exploring Facial Gender Affirmation Surgery

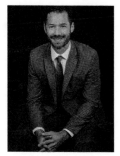

Michael T. Somenek, MD
Editor

Gender dysphoria (formerly gender identity disorder) is defined by strong, persistent feelings of identification with the opposite gender and discomfort with one's own assigned sex that results in significant distress or impairment. With the transgender population now exceeding 25 million globally, there has been an increasing need to provide gender affirming care. This increased awareness looks to address gender dysphoria in a comprehensive manner, which encompasses the spectrum from mental health, hormone replacement, and surgical intervention.

We formed a comprehensive collaboration of experts around the world to thoroughly describe and explain to surgeons the processes that are undertaken to assist individuals in making a successful transition. Our intention is to focus on the intricacies of surgical and medical interventions with the ultimate goal of helping individuals transition to their true gender. It is important to note that transgender individuals are forty times more likely to commit suicide than the general population. With proper treatment, however, gender dysphoric patients have an improved quality of life and demonstrate decreased psychosocial sequelae. Because of this, it is imperative as health care providers to ensure a comprehensive, high-quality care plan. To be able to do that, we need to ensure that physicians offering transgender care are appropriately trained and have the tools to implement adequate care.

I am honored to be part of the advancement of transgender medicine and feel that this publication provides a thorough discussion on important topics to empower physicians to provide the best care possible for this patient population. Continued enhancement in education and awareness will allow for improved multidisciplinary teams to address gender affirmation. I hope you find this educational, and more importantly, an insightful exploration into this incredible field.

Michael T. Somenek, MD
SomenekMD-
Advanced Facial Plastic Surgery
2440 M Street NW
Suite 507
Washington, DC 20037, USA

E-mail address:
drsomenek@somenekmd.com

Facial Plast Surg Clin N Am 27 (2019) xi
https://doi.org/10.1016/j.fsc.2019.02.001
1064-7406/19/© 2019 Published by Elsevier Inc.

Gender-related Facial Analysis

Chrisovalantis Lakhiani, MD[a], Michael T. Somenek, MD[b],*

KEYWORDS

• Gender • Face • Facial • analysis • Dysphoria

KEY POINTS

- There exist several known anthropometric differences between the male and female facial skeleton and soft tissues.
- The use of facial canons is not practical, and often inappropriate for analyzing morphologic differences of sex.
- A standardized system should be used for approaching facial analysis for gender dysphoric patients.

INTRODUCTION

Increasingly in the United States, gender dysphoria is being recognized by the surgical community, and transgender individuals are afforded the ability to undergo gender affirmation surgery. Current estimates for male-to-female transgenderism range from 1 in 11,900 to 1 in 45,000 for male-to-female individuals, and 1 in 30,400 to 1 in 200,000 for female-to-male individuals according to the World Professional Association for Transgender Health.[1] Still other scholars suggest that the prevalence of transgenderism is likely much higher.[1]

Although gender affirmation surgery has long been considered in the surgical literature, there is comparatively little describing morphologic differences between the feminine and masculine faces, and how to achieve them. The increasing prevalence of gender affirmation surgery reveals a shift in therapeutic treatments for gender dysphoria from being focused on the genitalia as the location of bodily sex toward an understanding of sex as a product of social recognition.[2] In a study by Ainsworth and Spiegel,[3] it was shown that the mental health quality of life for male-to-female individuals was diminished compared with the baseline population. However, performance of gender affirmation surgery resulted in a return of mental health quality of life to mean population levels. In addition, despite challenges associated with this surgery,[4] patient satisfaction levels following feminization of the male face are generally very high.[5,6]

Nevertheless, although aesthetic considerations for female facial morphology have been well described, the characteristics that allow a face to be recognized as decidedly masculine or feminine are more difficult to describe and not able to be recognized as a function of external influence (eg, gravity, sunlight). Often, surgeons are forced to use proportions of facial harmony that may be insufficient to achieve the patient goal, or inappropriate to use at all. This article provides a systematic method of facial analysis for gender dysphoric patients seeking facial affirmation surgery and elucidates critical areas that should be addressed with each patient so that the surgical plan and expectations can be discussed preoperatively.

BACKGROUND

The Greco-Roman artists sought to capture and numerically define the ideal form of the human

Disclosure: The authors have nothing to disclose.
[a] MedStar Georgetown University Hospital, 3800 Reservoir Road, Washington, DC 20007, USA; [b] Advanced Facial Plastic Surgery, 2440 M Street Northwest #507, Washington, DC 20037, USA
* Corresponding author.
E-mail address: drsomenek@somenekmd.com

Facial Plast Surg Clin N Am 27 (2019) 171–177
https://doi.org/10.1016/j.fsc.2019.01.006

figure. These forms have come to be known as artistic (sometimes divine) canons, or rules of simple proportions to describe the ideal human form. The canons of facial proportion evolved with the use of Pythagorean mathematics, the best known of which is the so-called golden proportion (1.618). The use of these canons was revived by Renaissance and neoclassical artists, including Albrecht Durer and Leonardo da Vinci. From these artists, several new canons were introduced, including division of the head and face into equal halves, thirds, or fourths, or vertically into equal fifths.[7,8]

What is currently known of the neoclassical canons is from the remnants of much larger bodies of work in artistic experimentation. That is, the intention of these artists was never to describe the typical or normal morphologic appearance of the human face. The growth of anthropometrics in the nineteenth and twentieth centuries afforded scientists the ability to confirm the reliability of the classical canons. The findings were that some of these familiar canons, such as the 3-part and 4-part horizontal divisions, do not exist in nature,[7,8] whereas others represent only a small fraction of natural variation[9] (**Fig. 1**).

The work of anthropometrists such as Leslie Farkas has offered insight into the diversity of human facial morphology. There are notable differences in morphology depending on race, ethnicity, age, and sex. Although it is established that concepts of fashion and beauty may vary by culture, there are generally distinct differences in facial sexual characteristics for any race or ethnicity. It is therefore important for surgeons to familiarize themselves with the anthropometric normative values for the population they are serving. Because a complete discussion of facial sexual dimorphism for all races or ethnicities is outside the scope of this article, this discussion is limited to the white population.

FACIAL ANALYSIS

In general, the male skull is larger, with an endocranial capacity approximately 200 g greater than that of the female, and is usually less round.[8,9] The female skull differs from the male in that it is has more pronounced zygomatic prominences leading to a pointed chin, creating a heart shape, compared with the squarer male skeleton.[10]

It is useful when analyzing the face in preparation for a masculinization or feminization procedure to divide the face into thirds and proceed using a top-to-bottom method. Thus, it is divided into the upper third (forehead region, brow), middle third (orbit, nose, cheeks), and lower third (lips, mandibular width, chin). Skeletal and soft tissue differences are each described for the anatomic subunit when appropriate.

Summaries of the differences between the male and female face and facial skeleton are provided in **Tables 1–3**.

UPPER THIRD

Analysis of the upper third of the face should include evaluation of the hairline shape, forehead length, forehead convexity, supraorbital bossing, glabella, nasofrontal angle, and brow position (see **Table 1**).

The feminine hairline is generally full and smooth contoured. In contrast, the male hairline may be receding and possess a so-called widow's peak or M-shaped hairline. There is generally a shorter distance from nasion to hairline in the female face by approximately 1 cm (5 cm in women, 6 cm in men).[10,11]

The supraorbital ridge is generally more pronounced in the male face, and there is a less steep slant from the supraorbital ridge to the vertex.[6,9,12] In contrast with the female forehead, which possesses a smooth convexity from the orbit to

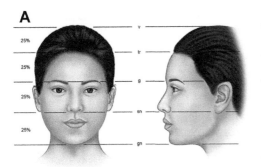
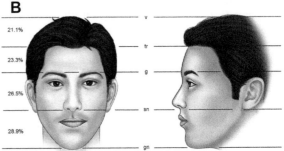

Fig. 1. The neoclassical canons of facial proportion have often been used as an adjunct to modern facial analysis (*A*, female; *B*, male). Nevertheless, the fallacy of these canons in restoring gender-related facial proportions is shown here, because normal anthropometric measurements are different.

Table 1
Upper third

Upper Third	Female	Male
Hairline shape	Smooth	M shaped
Nasion-trichion distance	Shorter than in men	High
Forehead convexity	Less convex, sloping	Flat or convex
Supraorbital bossing	Minimal or absent	Pronounced
Nasofrontal angle	Obtuse	Acute
Glabella	Less protruding	Wider, more protruding
Brow position	Above the supraorbital rim, raised at the lateral third	At the level of the supraorbital rim

vertex, the male forehead displays supraorbital bossing with a prominent anterior convexity to the forehead. Frontal sinus development contributes to greater convexity of the medial forehead in men, which leads to a discontinuous curvature compared with the female skull. Contrastingly, in women supraorbital bossing is considerably less, or minimal. The forehead is less flat, with a generally continuous mild curvature that continues to the vertex.[6,13]

In men, the medial supraorbital ridge blends into the glabella. Thus, men generally have a greater glabellar projection than women and this is considered more masculine.[10] However, the range of glabellar variation is much wider than that of the ridges.[9] More important in this region is attention to the nasofrontal angle, which is more acute in men and more obtuse in women.[14] Importantly, the nasoglabellar region represents the transition between the nose and forehead, and should be considered as an entity for affording facial harmony between upper and middle thirds during surgical planning.[15]

The female brow is club shaped medially, starts at or below the rim, then arches laterally to where it peaks at the lateral third. The most lateral portion of the female brow lies 1 to 2 mm above the medial aspect of the brow, and the entire brow lies at or above the superior orbital rim.[10] In contrast, the male brow tends to be thick, straighter, and tends to lie at the level of the superior orbital rim.[14,15] As in cis-gendered women, transgender women may also apply makeup or tattooing to enhance the shape or thickness of the brow. This makeup must also be noted when considering altering the shape or position of the brow (**Fig. 2**).

MIDDLE THIRD

Analysis of the middle third should include examination of the orbita and periorbital tissue, nose (with special notice of the nasal dorsum, tip, and alar base width), zygomatic width, and zygomatic prominence.

The female orbital height is less than that of men; however, the orbita are generally larger.[9] The upper and lateral portions of the orbital rims are less pronounced than in men.[16] The male upper eyelid crease is generally positioned lower, with a minimum of 8 mm above the lid margin, compared with a maximum of 12 mm for women. The male upper lid also appears fuller, with less pretarsal show.[10] The canthal tilt is subtly more positive in women.[8,10] In contradistinction to the upper lid, there are no significant differences in the lower eyelids of men and women. Spiegel makes note of the

Table 2
Middle third

Middle Third	Female	Male
Orbits	Wider, slight positive tilt	Narrower, neutral tilt
Zygomatic width	Slightly less wide	Wider
Zygomatic prominence	More prominent	Less prominent
Cheek hollowing	Varies by culture	Varies by culture
Nasal dorsum	Straight or slightly concave	Straight or dorsal hump
Alar base width	Much narrower	Wide

Table 3
Lower third

Lower Third	Female	Male
Lips	Greater vermilion show	Less vermilion show, greater cutaneous portion
Mandibular width	Narrower than zygomatic width	As wide as zygomatic width
Gonial angle	More obtuse	More acute
Chin	Trapezoidal, shorter	Square, longer

increased periorbital soft tissue luminance seen in women, likely caused by decreased dermal thickness, and suggests this be addressed as well.[17] The overall appearance is more youthful or cherubic, with larger orbita relative to facial volume and a less sunken appearance.

As previously noted, the nose has a more acute glabellar angle in men than in women.[6,7,9,13] Male nasal bones are generally larger and tend to meet in the midline at a sharper angle.[9,18] The nasal aperture in men is higher and narrower, with sharp rather than rounded margins. Thus, the male nose is somewhat square at the base with a more pronounced dorsal prominence. In contrast, female noses are smaller and shorter; they have narrower bridges and narrow alar bases, with a more obtuse nasolabial angle.[14,18] The male nose may have a dorsal hump or straight dorsum with very little supratip break, whereas the female nose is considered attractive if it shows a straight or mildly concave dorsum with an accented tip.[13,18] The male nose has a slightly wider nasal root than the female nose and a somewhat wider alar width. However, there is a significantly large difference between labial insertions of the alar base in men compared with women.[7] The nasal width to lip ratio is thus larger in men than in women.

The cheek bones are heavier in men, with a flatter convexity. Contrastingly, they are lighter but also more prominent in women.[9,12,14] Often, this is accentuated with some cheek hollowing in the submalar region. Increasing the width of the zygomatic complex creates more roundness of the facial contours and allows the orbits to appear larger.[12] Although interzygomatic distance is generally larger in men, the zygomatic prominence is generally more anterior in women. In addition, there is a significantly greater fullness in the maxilla relative to the mandible in women, which lends a heart-shaped appearance to the face[8] (**Fig. 3**).

LOWER THIRD

Analysis of the lower third should include examination of vermilion show and fullness, mandibular width, gonial angle, chin shape, chin height, and chin width.

Female upper lips are fuller and shorter with a good show of the vermilion and a well-formed Cupid's bow.[14] The upper lip is shorter and wider than in men. The vermilion and cutaneous portions of the lower lip in women are about equal in thickness, whereas in men the vermilion portion tends to be thinner than the cutaneous segment.[8] In

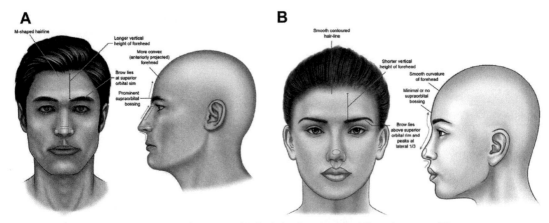

Fig. 2. The key differences between the upper third of the face in men (*A*) and women (*B*).

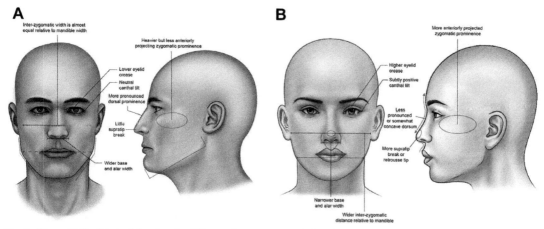

Fig. 3. The middle third of the face is different between men (*A*) and women (*B*) in the orbital, periorbital tissue quality, nasofrontal angle, nasal dorsum, tip, and base width, as well as the zygomatic prominences.

trans women, makeup or fillers may be used to accentuate lip fullness, and these should be noted as well when considering procedures to increase vermilion show.

The mandible in men is larger and thicker, with greater mandibular body height, especially at the symphysis. The male mandible is often heavier and taller, with a greater vertical height to the chin than in women.[9] In addition, men have more mandibular flare caused by mandibular attachments, resulting in a wider jaw.[12] The overall appearance in men is thus of a square or heavy-set jaw with a taller chin.

The mandibular angle should be assessed for its definition and sharpness. Women generally have a softer mandibular angle. The mandibular angle is generally less than 125° in both sexes; however, women tend to have a more obtuse angle than men by approximately 2.7°,[9,12] which creates a softer transition from the mandibular body to ramus, and a narrower mandibular width.

The chin and lower jaw is usually longer in men by as much as 20% and is often, but not always, more prominent in profile.[14] It is more trapezoidal, rather than rectangular in women than inn men.[12] In men, the shape is squarer because of bilateral lateral mental eminences in the region of the canines, whereas women generally have a single median mental eminence, giving their chins a more rounded or pointed appearance.[6,8,13] Although the female chin is slightly posterior to the lower lip vermilion, it is considered masculine if the chin is in line with the lower lip vermilion, or even slightly anterior to this.

When considering nasal-lip-chin relationships, it is important to also examine the patient's occlusion. This examination should include dentition, occlusal plane, and prior use of orthodontia. The use of orthodontia may mask a nonharmonious nasal-lip-chin relationship. A patient with class II malocclusion may have a retrodisplaced or micrognathic chin. This condition may be beneficial in the trans male-to-female population; however, in the trans female to male population, there may be a benefit to using a chin implant, corrective jaw surgery, and/or genioplasty to augment the chin and restore proper occlusion. Contrastingly, for those with class III occlusion, both trans-female and trans-male patients may benefit from corrective jaw surgery in order to restore normal occlusion; however, the mandibular setback or genioplasty for trans women should be greater than that for trans men (**Fig. 4**).

INTEGUMENT/SOFT TISSUE CONSIDERATIONS

It is worthwhile to mention the integumentary and soft tissue considerations between the male and female face. Clinicians should consider how patients wears their hair, the hairline (as discussed), presence of sideburns, brow thickness and position, eyelash length and volume, presence and distribution of facial hair, distribution of facial fat volume and fat compartments, as well as the overall quality and texture of the patient's skin.

Before undergoing surgery, trans-female patients may change their hairstyle to mask a high hairline by growing bangs or wearing a wig. The brow may be colored or tattooed in order to artificially create a higher and more arched brow as well. The eyelashes should be examined for length and volume, and the patient asked whether any products have been used to enhance the eyelash

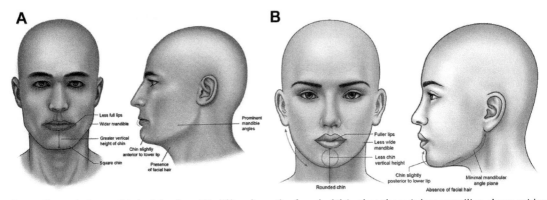

Fig. 4. The male lower third of the face (*A*) differs from the female (*B*) in that there is less vermilion show, wider mandibular width with greater mandibular angle flare, and a squarer chin with a taller vertical height.

length. The presence of facial hair is a decidedly masculine trait in Western cultures, and thus its presence warrants a discussion about hair removal strategies in trans male-to-female patients.

The male integument is 30 to 175 μm thicker than that of women, depending on the location being measured, and there is less subcutaneous fat, largely because of the presence of follicular units and adnexal structures under the influence of male hormones in the reticular dermis. The influence of estrogen contributes to the greater underlying subcutaneous fat, which leads to more fluid female contour, and less obvious muscular contraction during mimetic movements.[5,9] In addition, there exists some debate in the literature regarding the degree to which the sexes age and soft tissue descent occurs. Descent of the soft tissue may lead to a masculinized appearance of the female form. This is primarily due to descent of the brow and midface, a depressed canthal tilt, and squaring of the jaw. In these instances, a discussion of soft tissue rejuvenation procedures may be warranted, because the results of skeletal correction may not be as visibly appreciated.

SUMMARY

There exist several known anthropometric differences between the male and female facial skeleton and soft tissues. In general, the female face is less robust, rounder or heart shaped, with a shorter forehead, no supraorbital bossing, a smaller nose, more pronounced zygomatic prominences, fuller lips, a smaller mandibular width, and a more tapered chin. A method for analyzing these differences is critical for offering facial gender confirming surgery to gender dysphoric patients, for preoperative planning as well as for setting postoperative expectations.

REFERENCES

1. Coleman E, Bockting W, Cohen-Kettenis P, et al. Standards of care of the health of transsexual, transgender, and gender-nonconforming people. Int J Transgend 2011;13:165–232.
2. Plemons E. Formations of femininity: science and aesthetics in facial feminization surgery. Med Anthropol 2017;36(7):629–41.
3. Ainsworth TA, Spiegel JH. Quality of life of individuals with and without facial feminization surgery or gender reassignment surgery. Qual Life Res 2010;19(7):1019–24.
4. Spiegel JH. Challenges in care of the transgender patient seeking facial feminization surgery. Facial Plast Surg Clin North Am 2008;16(2):233–8. viii.
5. Raffaini M, Magri AS, Agostini T. Full facial feminization surgery: patient satisfaction assessment based on 180 procedures involving 33 consecutive patients. Plast Reconstr Surg 2016;137(2):438–48.
6. Ousterhout DK. Feminization of the forehead: contour changing to improve female aesthetics. Plast Reconstr Surg 1987;79(5):701–11.
7. Farkas LG. Anthropometry of the head and face. New York: Raven Press; 1994.
8. Ousterhout DK. Aesthetic contouring of the craniofacial skeleton. Boston: Little, Brown; 1991.
9. Hage JJ, Becking AG, de Graaf F, et al. Gender confirming facial surgery: considerations on the masculinity and femininity of faces. Plast Reconstr Surg 1997;99(7):1799–807.
10. Sedgh J. The aesthetics of the upper face and brow: male and female differences. Facial Plast Surg 2018;34(2):114–8.
11. Cho SW, Jin HR. Feminization of the forehead in a transgender: frontal sinus reshaping combined with brow lift and hairline lowering. Aesthetic Plast Surg 2012;36(5):1207–10.

12. Becking AG, Tuinzing DB, Hage JJ, et al. Transgender feminization of the facial skeleton. Clin Plast Surg 2007;34(3):557–64.

13. Dempf R, Eckert AW. Contouring the forehead and rhinoplasty in the feminization of the face in male-to-female transsexuals. J Craniomaxillofac Surg 2010;38(6):416–22.

14. Altman K. Facial fominization surgery: current state of the art. Int J Oral Maxillofac Surg 2012;41(8):885–94.

15. Capitan L, Simon D, Kaye K, et al. Facial feminization surgery: the forehead. Surgical techniques and analysis of results. Plast Reconstr Surg 2014; 134(4):609–19.

16. Lundgren TK, Farnebo F. Midface osteotomies for feminization of the facial skeleton. Plast Reconstr Surg Glob Open 2017;5(1):e1210.

17. Spiegel JH. Facial determinants of female gender and feminizing forehead cranioplasty. Laryngoscope 2011;121(2):250–61.

18. Nouraei SA, Randhawa P, Andrews P, et al. The role of nasal feminization rhinoplasty in male-to-female gender reassignment. Arch Facial Plast Surg 2007; 9(5):318–20.

Hormonal, Medical, and Nonsurgical Aspects of Gender Affirmation

Ronni Hayon, MD[a],*, Kristin Stevenson, MD[b]

KEYWORDS

- Transgender • Gender affirmation • Cultural competency • Hormonal therapy

KEY POINTS

- Transgender people have health needs that are unique and individual and experience significant health disparities.
- Creating a safe and welcoming clinical environment involves aspects of physical environment, interpersonal communication, customer service, the electronic health record, and institutional support.
- Gender-affirming treatment with medications and/or surgery should be individualized.

INTRODUCTION

Although the acronym LGBTQ is often used as a catchall label for sexual and gender minorities, the groups included under the umbrella of that acronym—lesbian, gay, bisexual, transgender, queer/questioning—have unique and individual health needs. In this section, the authors explore health care needs and issues that are unique to transgender people.

One of the cornerstones of providing competent care to transgender people is a thorough understanding of common terminology used in conversations about sex and gender. Even physicians often conflate these 2 concepts. The following are the high-yield terms and concepts:

- *Biological sex* is composed of genotype and phenotype (chromosomes, genitalia, etc.). Although most often we think of sex as a binary (male and female), there actually is a spectrum of biological sex (XX, XY, XO, XXY, XYY, mosaicism, etc).
- *Gender*, on the other hand, is the set of roles, activities, expectations, and behaviors assigned to women and men by society. Gender is defined by culture and historical period and is thus not immutable.
- *Gender identity* is our innermost sense of whether we are male, female, both, or neither. This can change over time and can only be self-identified by an individual.
- *Transgender* is a term that has multiple usages, some broad and some narrower. Broadly, "transgender" can describe anyone whose gender identity or expression falls outside of stereotypical "norms." More narrowly and more commonly, it is used to describe someone whose gender identity differs from their assigned sex at birth.

Disclosure Statement: No disclosure of any relationship with a commercial company that has a direct financial interest in subject matter or materials discussed in article or with a company making a competing product. This article does discuss off-label uses of medications.
[a] Department of Family Medicine and Community Health, University of Wisconsin, 1100 Delaplaine Ct., Madison, WI 53715, USA; [b] Department of Medicine, Division of Endocrinology, Diabetes & Metabolism, University of Wisconsin, Medical Foundation Centennial Building, Room 4170, 1685 Highland Avenue, Madison, WI 53705, USA
* Corresponding author.
E-mail address: Ronni.Hayon@fammed.wisc.edu

Facial Plast Surg Clin N Am 27 (2019) 179–190
https://doi.org/10.1016/j.fsc.2018.12.001

- *Sexual orientation* refers to romantic attraction. Our sexual orientation and our gender identity are separate, distinct parts of our overall identity, and may evolve or change over time. Being transgender does not imply any specific sexual orientation. Transgender people may identify as straight, gay, bisexual, or some other sexuality.
- *Gender dysphoria* is the term used in the Diagnostic and Statistical Manual of Mental Disorders (DSM) to describe the distress that is caused by the incongruence between an individual's gender identity and their sex assigned at birth. Not all transgender people experience gender dysphoria. The DSM clearly states that gender nonconformity itself is not a mental disorder. The critical element of gender dysphoria is the presence of clinically significant distress.[1]
- *Gender affirmation/transition* is the process of recognizing and accepting one's gender identity and then taking steps to express that gender identity. The primary foundation of transition-related care is individualization of care. There is no one right way to approach gender affirmation. The ultimate goal is increased congruence between internal gender identity and external expression and increased wellbeing. Not all transgender people want to undergo or are able to undergo medical or surgical therapy.

  Table 1 lists some common terms and definitions.

INCIDENCE/PREVALENCE

There are several challenges to collecting accurate data on the size of the transgender population. Examples of barriers include inconsistent collection of sexual orientation and gender identity (SOGI) data both at the clinic level and at the level of the national census, as well as reliance on data from gender-specialty centers, which vastly underestimates the transgender population because only a small percentage of gender-expansive patients will seek care at these centers. More recent studies using geographic or demographic sampling techniques have reported population-based estimates ranging from 0.33% to 1.6%, which are 10- to 100-fold higher than those reported in earlier studies.[2]

HEALTH DISPARITIES

Although there have been recent strides in increased awareness and acceptance, transgender people continue to experience significant

Table 1
Common terms and definitions

Term	Definition
Sex (n.)	Phenotypic and/or physiologic characteristics used to assign sex at birth (eg, chromosomes, hormones, and internal and external natal genitalia). Often referred to as "assigned sex at birth."
Sexual orientation (n.)	Term that refers to being romantically or sexually attracted to people of a specific gender (eg, a lesbian or gay man is someone who has attraction to a person of the same gender).
Gender (n.)	The set of roles, activities, expectations, and behaviors assigned to women and men by society, defined by culture and historical period.
Gender identity (n.)	One's innermost sense of self as male, female, both, or neither.
Gender expression (n.)	One's external expression of gender (eg, clothing, speech, mannerisms), which are conventionally considered masculine or feminine.
Transgender, gender-expansive, gender nonconforming (adj.)	Sometimes used as umbrella terms to describe anyone whose identity or behavior falls outside of stereotypical gender norms. More narrowly, refers to a person whose gender identity does not match their assigned birth sex.

(*continued on next page*)

Table 1
(continued)

Term	Definition
Nonbinary, gender queer (n.)	A gender identity or expression that is not strictly male or female.
Gender affirmation/ gender transition (n.)	The time period during which a person recognizes, accepts, and begins to live according to their gender identity, rather than the gender they were thought to be at birth. Each person's process is different and might include social, medical, or surgical components. (Older terms such as "sex-reassignment," "sex-change," or "cross-sex hormone therapy" can sometimes be perceived as pejorative and are falling out of usage.)
Cis-gender (adj.)	Refers to a person whose gender identity aligns with their assigned birth sex (ie, a nontransgender person).

minority stress and health disparities.[3,4] According to the most recent US Transgender Survey[4]

- When compared with the general population, transgender people experience higher rates of homelessness, poverty, psychological distress, suicidality, human immunodeficiency virus, bullying/mistreatment in school, and intimate partner violence.
- Transgender people of color experience even more profound and stark discrimination and disparities compared with white transgender people and the general US population.
- Thirty-three percent of respondents who saw a health care provider in the last year reported at least one negative experience related to gender identity (eg, refusal of treatment, verbal harassment, physical or sexual assault,

needing to teach health care provider about how to properly care for transgender people).
- Twenty-three percent of respondents did not see a doctor when they needed to because of fear of mistreatment.

Transgender people still struggle to get access to gender-affirming treatments and surgical procedures. Again, from the US Transgender Survey[4]

- Fifty-five percent of respondents who had sought coverage for transition-related surgery and 25% who had sought coverage for hormones in the past year were denied.[4]
- Twenty-one percent were covered by insurance for surgery but had no surgical providers in their network.[4]
- There is often a large gap between the percentage of transgender people who would like to have a gender-affirming surgery and the percentage of those who are actually able to access this care (**Figs. 1** and **2**).

There are an increasing number of studies that demonstrate that gender-affirming surgeries improve mental and physical health of transgender people.[5] The American Medical Association's 2016 policy recognizes that "medical and surgical treatments for gender dysphoria, as determined by shared decision making between the patient and physician, are medically necessary as outlined by generally-accepted standards of medical and surgical practice."[6] Multiple other professional organizations, including the World Professional Association for Transgender Health (WPATH), the American Psychological Association, the American Academy of Family Physicians, and the American College of Obstetricians and Gynecologists have issued similar statements. The idea that medical and surgical interventions are cosmetic rather than medically necessary is out of line with current medical recommendations.[5,7]

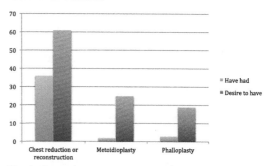

Fig. 1. Surgeries among transgender men. (*Data from* James SE, Herman JL, Rankin S, et al. The report of the 2015 U.S. transgender survey. Washington, DC: The National Center for Transgender Equality; 2016.)

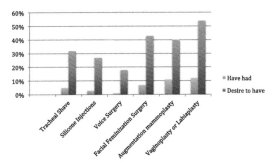

Fig. 2. Surgeries among transgender women. (*Data from* James SE, Herman JL, Rankin S, et al. The report of the 2015 U.S. transgender survey. Washington, DC: The National Center for Transgender Equality; 2016.)

These disparities and access gaps, along with the lack of in-network surgical providers who provide gender-affirming procedures, represent an opportunity for plastic surgeons to help improve access to this medically necessary care and reduce health disparities.

CREATING A WELCOMING ENVIRONMENT

The physical space of a clinic or hospital provides an important first impression for gender-expansive people seeking care. Often, patients will look for clues that a health care facility is a safe place for them to seek care.[8,9]

There are several improvements that can be implemented in the clinic or hospital environment that can create a culture of safety and welcome for transgender people:

- Window decals or stickers of the gay pride flag (rainbow) or transgender pride flag (5 horizontal stripes: light blue, pink, white, pink, and light blue) are signs of welcome to the LGBTQ community that, if placed on the front door or window, can be seen by patients as they first enter the clinic.
- Waiting room: display posters or artwork that represent LGBTQ people, have magazines or pamphlets that focus on LGBTQ issues available.
- Simply using the restroom can be a stressful and fraught experience for transgender patients. Making sure that there is a clearly marked single occupancy or gender-neutral restroom in the clinic/hospital that transgender people can access safely is an important aspect of creating a welcoming space.

VERBAL AND WRITTEN COMMUNICATION

Treating transgender patients with respect aligns with core principles of customer service and begins with a patient's first interaction with the registration desk. As with any patient encounter, maintaining privacy and avoiding collecting sensitive information in public areas are essential aspects of providing clinical care.[10]

Pronouns are words that we use in discourse to refer to others, such as she/her/hers and he/him/his. Some gender-expansive people may use gender-neutral pronouns such as they/them/their or ze/zir/zirself (eg, "Did you see the scarf they were wearing? They knitted it themselves." or "Did you see the scarf ze is wearing? Ze knitted it zirself."). Although it may seem grammatically incorrect or feel awkward at first, using correct pronouns is an essential part of providing appropriate care to gender-expansive patients because it validates gender identity and creates a therapeutic relationship. Using the wrong name or pronouns is known as "misgendering," and it is not only disrespectful and invalidating but can also lead to patients feeling unsafe in the clinical environment and avoiding care.[11]

Table 2 gives some examples of certain phrases to include (or avoid) during conversations with patients who are transgender.

Having intake forms that have LGBTQ-inclusive options and/or open-ended questions with blank spaces for patients to provide answers will increase patient comfort and inclusivity. Multiple organizations including the US Centers for Disease Control have endorsed a 2-step method for gathering gender identity data. The 2-question method uses multiple-choice questions and allows patients to self-report gender identity (ie, male, female, transgender, gender queer, additional gender identity, decline to state) as well as the sex assigned at birth (ie, male, female, intersex, decline to state). The 2-question approach has been shown to be acceptable to patients and increase response rates on questionnaires.[12]

THE ELECTRONIC HEALTH RECORD

In 2015, the Centers for Medicare and Medicaid Services and the Office of the National Coordinator for Health Information Technology ruled that in order to be certified for Stage 3 Meaningful Use, electronic health record (EHR) software must include sexual orientation and gender identity fields.[13]

Having accurate and complete SOGI data in the EHR is essential for fostering a clinical environment that is not stigmatizing or harmful for transgender people, for creating an accurate record of which organs a patient has so that their treating clinician can make accurate screening and treatment decisions, and also for building robust data sets for ongoing clinical research to assess health

Table 2
How to respond to common scenarios

Scenario	Language to Use	Language to Avoid
Patient arrives at registration desk	"How may I help you today?"	"How may I help you, sir/ma'am?"
Discrepancy between name given by patient and name on medical record	"Is it possible your chart is under a different name?"	"What's your real name?"
Unsure how to address a patient	"What name and pronouns do you use?"	Using name/pronouns you assume to be correct
Collecting SO/GI information	"Because many of our patients are affected by gender issues, I ask everyone these questions about sexual orientation and gender identity."	"Are you male or female?" "You look like a real woman/man! I never would have guessed!"
Staff member uses wrong name/pronouns	"I'm very sorry that I used the wrong name/pronoun."	"I just can't remember to use that name/pronoun." "You don't look male/female, so you can't blame me for using that name/pronoun."
Patient presents for services not related to gender	Address the clinical issue at hand	Inquiring about gender transition, what organs/genitals someone has, or what surgeries they have had

Adapted from Reisner S. Meeting the health care needs of transgender people. Available at: http://www.lgbthealtheducation.org/wp-content/uploads/Sari-slides_final1.pdf. Accessed May 30, 2018; with permission.

disparities and interventions that can benefit the LGBTQ population.[13]

Transgender people have unique needs in regard to how demographic information and medical information are recorded and displayed in the EHR. Demographic information includes data such as name, SOGI information, and pronouns. Pertinent medical information includes medications used, which organs have been surgically enhanced or removed, and which organs remain. The EHR can often obscure this information by prepopulating note templates based on the sex noted in the chart or by not clearly guiding users to use appropriate names and pronouns. The WPATH EMR Working Group has published recommendations for how to use the EHR in a way that fosters patient comfort as well as accurate medical information for the treating clinician.[14] Key recommendations on EHR use from WPATH are as follows:

- The system should include preferred name, gender identity, and preferred pronouns in demographic data.
- Provide a way to document a patient's medical history and current anatomy inventory, which is uncoupled from the demographic information about gender identity, assigned sex, or pronouns.

- The process of transitioning from one name, anatomic inventory, and/or sex should be smooth.
- The EHR should include an easily recognizable alert to notify users of a patient's proper name and pronouns (eg, a flag in the banner at the top of the screen).

INSTITUTIONAL SUPPORT

In addition to individual interactions that foster a welcoming environment, there are several institution-level interventions that play a crucial role in creating a positive and safe experience for transgender patients[8–10]:

- Nondiscrimination statements: create, post, and enforce a nondiscrimination policy that includes "gender identity and expression." Examples of such policies from health care organizations can be found here: https://www.hrc.org/hei/patient-non-discrimination-sample-policies.
- Visitation policy: creating a written policy on visitation rights and medical decision-making that explicitly includes partners, children, and family of choice for LGBTQ patients.
- Training: ongoing annual training for all staff and prompt training for new staff to maintain

competency of all employees who interact with transgender patients either in person or on the phone.

- The Human Rights Campaign has created an online resource, the Healthcare Equality Index (HEI), which health care organizations may use to evaluate the inclusiveness and patient centeredness of their policies and practices. The HEI Website also houses several resources for health care systems to create transgender-affirming hospital policies and a transinclusive workplace (https://www.hrc.org/hei).

RESOURCES FOR FURTHER READING

UCSF Center of Excellence for Transgender Health
- http://www.transhealth.ucsf.edu
- Primary care protocols for practitioners caring for gender-expansive patients
- Online learning center

World Professional Association for Transgender Health
- http://www.wpath.org/
- Interdisciplinary professional and educational organization devoted to transgender health
- Mission: to promote evidence-based care, education, research, advocacy, public policy, and respect in transgender health.
- Free download of standards of care manual
- Conferences, symposia, and trainings

National LGBT Health Education Center
- https://www.lgbthealtheducation.org
- Free online learning modules and resources
- Also offers consultation to health care organizations with the goal of optimizing quality and cost-effective health care for lesbian, gay, bisexual, and transgender (LGBT) people.

Gay and Lesbian Medical Association Transgender Health Resources
- http://www.glma.org/
- Online learning modules and glossaries
- Online referral directory for patients

National Center for Transgender Equality
- http://transequality.org/
- Social justice organization dedicated to advancing the equality of transgender people through advocacy, collaboration, and empowerment

Philadelphia Trans Health Conference
- https://www.mazzonicenter.org/trans-health
- Yearly conference that includes a Professional Development track for medical providers, behavioral health professionals, and lawyers.

Centers for Disease Control

- https://www.cdc.gov/lgbthealth/transgender.htm
- Resources for health care providers and patients

Human Rights Campaign—Healthcare Equality Index
- http://www.hrc.org/hei
- Resources available on nondiscrimination and staff training, patient services and support, employee benefits and policies, and patient and community engagement and resources for Veterans Affairs Medical Facilities.

Hormone Therapy for Transgender Individuals

The overall goal of treatment of gender dysphoria is to reduce the distress caused by the discrepancy between a person's gender identity and their sex assigned at birth. Hormonal treatment of gender dysphoria primarily works to address the incongruence in secondary sex characteristics. Feminizing or masculinizing hormone therapy is a medically necessary intervention for many individuals with gender dysphoria.[15,16] Accordingly, WPATH, the Endocrine Society, and UCSF's Center of Excellence for Transgender Health have published guidelines that include recommendations on the medical management of gender dysphoria that are widely used by specialists in transgender health care.[16–18]

The 2 key components of hormonal treatment of gender dysphoria are reducing endogenous sex hormone levels as determined by the individual's sex assigned at birth and replacing endogenous sex hormones to normal levels consistent with the individual's affirmed gender.[18] The physical changes caused by gender-affirming hormone therapy are usually associated with improved mental well-being.[19,20]

Criteria for Treatment

Criteria for initiation of gender-affirming hormone therapy as proposed by WPATH include the following[16]:

1. Persistent, well-documented gender dysphoria/gender incongruence.
2. Capacity to make a fully informed decision and to consent for treatment.
3. Age of majority in a given country.
4. Mental health concerns, if present, must be reasonably well controlled.

Endocrine Society guidelines are in agreement with these criteria; in addition, they recommend that clinicians evaluate and address medical conditions that could be exacerbated by hormone therapy before initiation of treatment.[18].

Pretreatment Counseling and Evaluation

Treatment goals
Hormone therapy and goals of treatment must be individualized. Some individuals may seek maximum feminization or masculinization, whereas others may be satisfied with minimization of their existing secondary sex characteristics.[16,21]

Risk assessment
The patient's individual risk factors for hormone-related adverse events should be evaluated, and they should also undergo appropriate screening tests for conditions affected by hormone therapy, depending on their age and risk profile.[16] The presence of other comorbid medical conditions must also be taken into account when assessing the individualized risk/benefit ratio.[16] To that end, it is recommended that transgender patients undergo a comprehensive history and physical examination, including screening for hepatic and renal dysfunction, hyperlipidemia, and diabetes before initiation of hormone therapy.[16,18,22]

Fertility considerations
It is important that transgender patients be counseled regarding options for fertility preservation before the initiation of hormone therapy.[16,18] Although there are some case reports of transgender people using their natal gametes for reproduction after long-term use of gender-affirming hormones, the long-term effects of these medications on fertility are not well-known.[18,23–25]

Feminizing Hormone Therapy

Estrogen therapy
There are several commercially available estrogen formulations available (**Table 3**). The recommended treatment is 17β-estradiol as an oral, sublingual, transdermal, or occasionally injectable preparation.[18,26] Current guidelines do not specify a preferential order in which these therapies should be chosen, primarily because data comparing them are lacking.[18,26] However, there is some evidence that oral preparations may be more thrombogenic due to "first-pass" metabolism in the liver, and therefore transdermal, injectable, and sublingual preparations that bypass this route may be advantageous in older patients or those otherwise at increased risk for thromboembolic events.[18,26,27]

Generally, use of injectable estradiol is less common and is more often used in patients who do not achieve hormonal goals despite using the maximum recommended dose of either oral or transdermal estrogen preparations.[26] Oral ethinyl estradiol in particular has been shown to carry a higher risk of venous thromboembolism, and therefore its use is not recommended.[27] Conjugated and synthetic estrogens cannot be monitored through blood tests and therefore are of limited use.[26]

Androgen suppression
Treatment with estrogen alone is usually insufficient to reduce testosterone levels to the physiologic range for cis women, so transgender women generally require adjunctive antiandrogen therapy.[18,28] The most commonly used

Table 3
Hormone regimens for transgender women

Medication	Route	Recommended Dose	Considerations
Estrogen	Oral	2–6 mg/d	Higher thromboembolic risk
	Transdermal	0.025–0.2 mg/24 h once or twice weekly	Possible skin reaction, more constant blood levels
	Parenteral	5–20 mg IM every 2 wk or 2–10 mg IM weekly	
Cyproterone acetate	Oral	25–50 mg/d	Not available in United States, possible liver toxicity
GnRH agonists	Parenteral	Leuprolide: 3.75 mg SC monthly or 11.25 mg SC every 3 mo Goserelin acetate: 3–6 mg SC monthly or 10–8 mg SC every 3 mo	Expensive
Spironolactone	Oral	100–300 mg/d	

Abbreviations: GnRH, gonadotropin-releasing hormone; IM, intramuscular; SC, subcutaneous.
Data from Refs.[18,26,30]

Table 4
Hormone regimens for transgender men

Medication	Route	Recommended Dose	Considerations
Testosterone	Transdermal		
	Patch	2.5–7.5 mg/d	Possible skin irritation
	Gel	50–100 mg/d	Mimics physiologic secretion, possible transfer to partners
	Parenteral		
	Enanthate, cypionate	100–250 mg IM (SC) every 2–4 wk or 50–100 mg IM weekly	Supraphysiologic levels after injection, with decline before next administration
	Undecanoate	1000 mg every 12 wk	More stable blood levels

Data from Refs.[18,23,26,41]

antiandrogen therapies include spironolactone, cyproterone acetate, and gonadotropin-releasing hormone (GnRH) agonists (**Table 4**). Spironolactone inhibits testosterone secretion, blocks androgen receptor binding, and may also have estrogenic activity.[18,26] Cyproterone acetate is a synthetic progestogen compound with antiandrogen properties widely used in Europe but is not available in the United States due to concerns for liver toxicity.[29] GnRH agonists are used to inhibit gonadotropin secretion and thereby induce profound suppression of testosterone secretion; they are given as long-acting injections and are highly effective, however their cost can be prohibitive.[16,29]

The 5α-reductase inhibitors are also sometimes used. These medications block conversion of testosterone to the potent androgen dihydrotestosterone. Although Endocrine Society guidelines do not specifically recommend their use because they do not reduce testosterone levels and may be associated with adverse effects,[18,29,30] other groups including UCSF and WPATH note that they may be beneficial especially for individuals unable to tolerate or with contraindications to spironolactone or for those with persistently virilized features despite complete androgen blockade.[16,31]

Other therapies

Progestins have sometimes been used for the treatment of transgender women. Reports of possibly improved breast development have been associated with their use. However, they have not been well studied as part of a gender-affirming hormone regimen, and overall there is little data to either support or dissuade their use. Because of this lack of data and concerns regarding possibly increased risk of breast cancer and cardiovascular disease (based on data in menopausal and postmenopausal

nontransgender patients), Endocrine Society and WPATH guidelines do not specifically recommend their use.[16,18,26,29] However, other groups including UCSF note that the risk in transgender patients is likely minimal-to-absent.

Clinical outcomes

Initial physical changes include decreased body hair, decreased libido and spontaneous erections, decreased lean muscle mass and strength, decreased oiliness of the skin, increased weight, and redistribution of fat mass with an increase in subcutaneous fat.[18,32,33] Long-term treatment will result in atrophy of the prostate and testes.[18,33] Facial hair is also reduced with hormonal therapy; however, elimination is difficult to achieve. Some patients may choose to pursue additional measures such as electrolysis or laser treatments to achieve their desired appearance.[26,33] Breast development begins within the first 3 to 6 months of treatment and is typically at its maximum by 2 years.[29,33] Approximately 50% of transgender women will be dissatisfied with the breast growth attained from hormone therapy alone, prompting some to seek gender affirming surgeries.[32]

Monitoring

Transgender women should be monitored closely following initiation of hormone therapy. Current guidelines advise regular clinical evaluations and assessment for physical changes of feminization/masculinization and for possible adverse effects from hormone therapy, as well as laboratory monitoring of sex steroid hormone levels every 3 months during the first year of treatment and then 1 to 2 times yearly.[18]

A key issue in monitoring transgender women is to avoid supraphysiologic levels of estrogen that may lead to increased risk of adverse events. Goal hormone levels are within the physiologic cis-female range. This corresponds with serum testosterone levels less than 50 ng/dL and serum estradiol levels that should not exceed the peak physiologic range of 100 to 200 pg/mL.[16,18] For patients on spironolactone, it is also recommended to monitor serum electrolytes.[18]

Pituitary lactotroph cells contain estrogen receptors, and thus up to 20% of patients receiving estrogen therapy may have increased prolactin levels while on gender-affirming medications.[16,18,29] The risk of development of prolactinoma is thought to be very low; however, some current guidelines advise monitoring prolactin levels at baseline, annually during the transition period, and at least every 2 years thereafter.[18] Other guidelines recommend checking prolactin levels only if symptoms of prolactinoma (visual symptoms, excessive galactorrhea, new onset headaches.[31]

Risks and adverse events

Venous thromboembolism (VTE) may be a serious complication in transgender women treated with estrogen. A 20-fold increase in venous thromboembolic events was seen in a study of Dutch transgender patients; however, this increased risk may have been related to the use of ethinyl estradiol, which carries an increased risk of VTE.[18,26,34] More recent studies have shown a lower risk of VTE.[35–37] Most recently, a large cohort study showed an increased risk of VTE and ischemic stroke with the use of gender-affirming hormones. Clot rates in trans women were about 5 times higher after two years of follow up when compared to cisgender men. Ischemic stroke risk in transgender women was approximately 10 times higher when compared to cisgender men, and about 4 times higher compared to cisgender women. Though this data suggests increased cardiovascular risks for transgender women, it is important to note that the actual number of events recorded in the study was 148 out of the 2,842 transgender women in the eight-year period of the study. While this new data should serve to underscore the importance of informed consent discussions and thoughtful consideration of which formulation of estrogen to use, it is important to note that for many transgender people, these medications are life-saving, and patients may decide that the associated risks are not high enough to dissuade them from starting gender affirming therapy.[38] Transdermal estrogen is recommended for older patients or those at increased risk of VTE due to avoidance of "first pass" metabolism and therefore reduced thrombogenicity, as discussed earlier. Note that guidelines recommend against screening for hereditary thrombophilia in most patients; however, it could be considered for those with a personal or family history of thromboembolic events.[16,18]

Overall, data regarding bone mineral density (BMD) and osteoporosis in transgender patients are limited. Estrogen has been shown to preserve BMD in patients who continue on therapy.[18,29] However, transgender patients who undergo gonadectomy and then choose to discontinue hormone therapy are clearly at increased risk for bone loss. Fracture data are not known for transgender patients, nor is it known whether to use sex assigned at birth or affirmed gender when estimating fracture risk.[18]

As described above, there is conflicting data regarding hormonal therapy in transgender women and cardiovascular risk. It is recommended that transgender women be assessed for cardiovascular risk factors with lipid panels and diabetes screening according to established guidelines.[18]

Masculinizing Hormone Therapy

Androgens

There are several androgen preparations available with demonstrated clinical efficacy (see **Fig. 1**). Testosterone is most often administered either parenterally or transdermally. Parenteral formulations include testosterone enanthate or cypionate, which can be injected intramuscularly every 1 to 2 weeks, and testosterone undecanoate, which may be given intramuscularly at longer intervals up to 10 to 12 weeks.[18,23,39]

Transdermal testosterone may be administered via gel or patch. Transdermal preparations may be associated with risk of skin irritation and risk of testosterone gel transfer to others. Short-term studies have shown no difference between parenteral or transdermal preparations with regard to body composition, metabolic parameters, safety, compliance, or satisfaction.[23,40]

Clinical outcomes

Testosterone therapy in transgender men results in clinical effects of virilization. During the first 1 to 6 months of treatment, expected changes include increased muscle mass, redistribution of fat mass, increased sexual desire, increased oiliness of skin, increased facial and body hair, and cessation of menses. Changes that may appear later (but still within the first year of treatment) include deepening of the voice, clitoromegaly, and sometimes male pattern hair loss.[18,23,32] It is important to note that height and bone structure are not altered by testosterone therapy.[23] In addition, testosterone therapy may decrease glandular activity of the breast but will not decrease breast size.[32]

Acne may be a significant undesired effect of testosterone therapy. The prevalence and severity of these lesions usually peaks by 6 months and tends to resolve in transgender men who continue therapy long-term.[23,41]

Monitoring

As with transgender women, transgender men should be monitored closely following initiation of treatment with regular clinical evaluations including assessment for physical changes of masculinization and possible adverse effects of hormone therapy, as well as regular laboratory monitoring.[16,18]

A major goal of monitoring treatment is to achieve testosterone levels in the normal cis-male range, which is assay dependent but typically between 320 and 1000 ng/dL.[18,28] Supraphysiologic levels of testosterone should be avoided because this may increase the risk of adverse reactions.

It is recommended that testosterone levels be monitored every 3 months until levels are in the normal physiologic cis-male range or for the first year of treatment (whichever is longer) and then 1 to 2 times annually thereafter. Current guidelines also recommend that hematocrit be monitored at baseline, every 3 months during first year of treatment and annually thereafter. When interpreting hematologic laboratory results, the "male" range should be used. Weight, blood pressure, and lipids should also be monitored at regular intervals.[16,18,39]

Risks and adverse events

A major concern with testosterone therapy has been the possibility of cardiovascular adverse events. Testosterone therapy in transgender men has been shown to result in a more atherogenic lipid profile with increased low-density lipoprotein and triglycerides and decreased high-density lipoprotein.[42] However, 2 meta-analyses did not show any increased incidence of cardiovascular events in patients on testosterone therapy,[43,44] and a long-term study in transgender men found no increased risk of cardiovascular mortality.[34] Current guidelines recommend that clinicians should screen for and manage cardiovascular risk factors as they emerge according to established screening guidelines.[16,18]

Testosterone therapy has been found to prevent bone loss in transgender men who have undergone gonadectomy.[45] However, some transgender men on hormone therapy do not maintain bone mass; this is thought to be related to low testosterone dosing and nonsuppressed luteinizing hormone concentrations, demonstrating the importance of adequate dosing of testosterone for maintenance of bone mass.[46] As with transgender women, transgender men who undergo gonadectomy and then stop testosterone therapy are at high risk for bone loss.[18]

Perioperative Concerns Related to Hormone Therapy

Timing of gender-affirming surgery

Current guidelines recommend that transgender patients use gender-affirming hormones for 1 year before gender-affirming surgery involving genitals or gonads.[16,18]

For transgender women, it is recommended that breast augmentation surgery be delayed until the patient has completed at least 2 years of estrogen therapy because breast development may continue throughout this period. However, hormone therapy is not a prerequisite for breast or chest surgery for transgender men or women.[16,18,22]

Risk of venous thromboembolism

Perioperative venous thromboembolism may be a risk in transgender women treated with estrogen, and surgical procedures and associated immobilization confer additional risk for thromboembolic events. Data on the incidence and risk of venous thromboembolism in transgender patients treated with estrogen undergoing surgery are limited. However, one review of 60 transgender patients undergoing gender-affirming surgery after 1 year of hormonal therapy did not report any venous thromboembolic events.[47]

Given the perceived increased risks, hormone therapy is frequently held perioperatively in transgender patients. However, there is currently minimal data to guide this decision. Some investigators suggest that estrogen therapy should be discontinued between 2 and 4 weeks before gender-affirming surgery, with resumption of therapy 3 to 4 weeks following surgery, or once patients are fully mobilized again.[32,36] It is common practice to temporarily interrupt hormone therapy for longer surgical procedures such as vaginoplasties, which also require modified bed rest for up to a week postoperatively. However, hormones may sometimes be continued for outpatient procedures or those that are completed in less than 4 to 5 hours. Current guidelines suggest that the surgeon and hormone-prescribing physician collaborate in making a decision about the use of hormones before and following surgery.[18]

REFERENCES

1. American Psychiatric Association. Diagnostic and statistical manual of mental disorders, 5th edition.

Arlington (VA): American Psychiatric Association; 2013. Available at: https://doi.org/10.1176/appi. books.9780890425596.744053.

2. Deutsch MB. Making it count: improving estimates of the size of transgender and gender nonconforming populations. LGBT Health 2016;3(3):181–5.

3. Valentine SE, Shipherd JC. A systematic review of social stress and mental health among transgender and gender non-conforming people in the United States. Clin Psychol Rev 2018. Available at: https://doi.org/10.1016/j.cpr.2018.03.003.

4. James SE, Herman JL, Rankin S, et al. The report of the 2015 U.S. transgender survey 2016. Available at: https://transequality.org/sites/default/files/docs/usts/USTS-Full-Report-Dec17.pdf. Accessed May 22, 2018.

5. Kuzon WM, Sluiter E, Gast KM. Exclusion of medically necessary gender-affirming surgery for America's Armed Services Veterans. AMA J Ethics 2018; 20(4):403–13.

6. American Medical Association. Clarification of medical necessity for treatment of gender dysphoria H-185.927 2016. Available at: https://policysearch. ama-assn.org/policyfinder/detail/H-185.927 sort% 3A?uri=%2FAMADoc%2FHOD-185.927.xml. Accessed June 4, 2018.

7. Bau I, Baker K. Legal and policy issues. In: Eckstrand KL, Ehrenfeld JM, editors. Bian, gay, bisexual, and transgender healthcare: a clinical guide to preventive, primary, and specialist care. Cham (Switzerland): Springer International; 2016. p. 421–40.

8. GLMA. Guidelines for care of lesbian, gay, bisexual, and transgender patients. 2006. Available at: http://www.glma.org/_data/n_0001/resources/live/Welcoming Environment.pdf. Accessed June 5, 2018.

9. Reisner S. Meeting the health care needs of transgender people. Available at: http://www. lgbthealtheducation.org/wp-content/uploads/Sari-slides_final1.pdf. Accessed May 30, 2018.

10. Sheedy CA. Clinic and intake forms. In: Eckstrand K, Ehrenfeld J, editors. Lesbian, gay, bisexual, and transgender healthcare: a clinical guide to preventive, primary and specialist care. Cham (Switzerland): Springer International; 2016. p. 175–211.

11. White Hughto JM, Rose AJ, Pachankis JE, et al. Barriers to gender transition-related healthcare: identifying underserved transgender adults in Massachusetts. Transgend Health 2017;2(1):107–18.

12. Tate CC, Ledbetter JN, Youssef CP. A two-question method for assessing gender categories in the social and medical sciences. J Sex Res 2013;50(8): 767–76.

13. Cahill SR, Baker K, Deutsch MB, et al. Inclusion of sexual orientation and gender identity in stage 3 meaningful use guidelines: a huge step forward for LGBT health. LGBT Health 2016;3(2):100–2.

14. Deutsch MB, Green J, Keatley J, et al. Electronic medical records and the transgender patient: recommendations from the World Professional Association for Transgender Health EMR Working Group. J Am Med Inform Assoc 2013;20(4): 700–3.

15. Newfield E, Hart S, Dibble S, et al. Female-to-male transgender quality of life. Qual Life Res 2006; 15(9):1447–57.

16. Coleman E, Bockting W, Botzer M, et al. Standards of care for the health of transsexual, transgender, and gender-nonconforming people, version 7. Int J Transgend 2012;13(4):165–232.

17. American College of Obstetricians and Gynecologists. Health care for transgender individuals. Obstet Gynecol 2011;118(6):1454–8.

18. Hembree WC, Cohen-Kettenis PT, Gooren L, et al. Endocrine treatment of gender-dysphoric/gender-incongruent persons: an endocrine society clinical practice guideline. J Clin Endocrinol Metab 2017; 102(11):3869–903.

19. Heylens G, Verroken C, De Cock S, et al. Effects of different steps in gender reassignment therapy on psychopathology: a prospective study of persons with a gender identity disorder. J Sex Med 2014; 11(1):119–26.

20. Costa R, Colizzi M. The effect of cross-sex hormonal treatment on gender dysphoria individuals' mental health: a systematic review. Neuropsychiatr Dis Treat 2016;12:1953–66.

21. Factor R, Rothblum E. Exploring gender identity and community among three groups of transgender individuals in the United States: MTSs, FTMs, and genderqueers. Health Sociol Rev 2008;17(3):235–53.

22. Meyer WJ, Webb A, Stuart CA, et al. Physical and hormonal evaluation of transsexual patients: a longitudinal study. Arch Sex Behav 1986;15(2):121–38.

23. Meriggiola MC, Gava G. Endocrine care of transpeople part I. A review of cross-sex hormonal treatments, outcomes and adverse effects in transmen. Clin Endocrinol (Oxf) 2015;83(5):597–606.

24. Light AD, Obedin-Maliver J, Sevelius JM, et al. Transgender men who experienced pregnancy after female-to-male gender transitioning. Obstet Gynecol 2014;124(6):1120–7.

25. De Roo C, Tilleman K, T'sjoen G, et al. Fertility options in transgender people Fertility options in transgender people. Int Rev Psychiatry 2016;28(1):112–9.

26. Knezevich EL, Viereck LK, Drincic AT. Medical management of adult transsexual persons. Pharmacotherapy 2012;32(1):54–66.

27. Toorians AWFT, Thomassen MCLGD, Zweegman S, et al. Venous thrombosis and changes of hemostatic variables during cross-sex hormone treatment in transsexual people. J Clin Endocrinol Metab 2003; 88(12):5723–9.

28. Gooren LJ, Giltay EJ, Bunck MC. Long-term treatment of transsexuals with cross-sex hormones: extensive personal experience. J Clin Endocrinol Metab 2008;93(1):19–25.

29. Meriggiola MC, Gava G. Endocrine care of transpeople part II. A review of cross-sex hormonal treatments, outcomes and adverse effects in transwomen. Clin Endocrinol (Oxf) 2015;83(5):607–15.

30. Chiriacò G, Cauci S, Mazzon G, et al. An observational retrospective evaluation of 79 young men with long-term adverse effects after use of finasteride against androgenetic alopecia. Andrology 2016;4(2):245–50.

31. UCSF. Guidelines for the primary and gender-affirming care of transgender and gender nonbinary people. 2nd edition. Dep Fam Community Med Cent Excell Transgender Heal; 2016. Available at: www.transhealth.ucsf.edu/guidelines.

32. Gooren L. Hormone treatment of the adult transsexual patient. Horm Res 2005;64(Suppl. 2):31–6.

33. Moore E, Wisniewski A, Dobs A. Endocrine treatment of transsexual people: A review of treatment regimens, outcomes, and adverse effects. J Clin Endocrinol Metab 2003;88(8):3467–73.

34. van Kesteren PJ, Asscheman H, Megens JA, et al. Mortality and morbidity in transsexual subjects treated with cross-sex hormones. Clin Endocrinol (Oxf) 1997;47(3):337–42.

35. Wierckx K, Van Caenegem E, Schreiner T, et al. Cross-sex hormone therapy in trans persons is safe and effective at short-time follow-up: results from the European network for the investigation of gender incongruence. J Sex Med 2014;11(8):1999–2011.

36. Asscheman H, T'Sjoen G, Lemaire A, et al. Venous thrombo-embolism as a complication of cross-sex hormone treatment of male-to-female transsexual subjects: a review. Andrologia 2014;46(7):791–5.

37. Righini M, Perrier A, De Moerloose P, et al. D-Dimer for venous thromboembolism diagnosis: 20 years later. J Thromb Haemost 2008;6(7):1059–71.

38. Getahun D, Nash R, Flanders WD, et al. Cross-sex hormones and acute cardiovascular events in transgender persons: a cohort study. Ann Intern Med 2018;169:205–13.

39. Bhasin S, Cunningham GR, Hayes FJ, et al. Testosterone therapy in adult men with androgen deficiency syndromes: an endocrine society clinical practice guideline. J Clin Endocrinol Metab 2006; 91(6):1995–2010.

40. Pelusi C, Costantino A, Martelli V, et al. Effects of three different testosterone formulations in female-to-male transsexual persons. J Sex Med 2014; 11(12):3002–11.

41. Wierckx K, Van de Peer F, Verhaeghe E, et al. Short- and long-term clinical skin effects of testosterone treatment in trans men. J Sex Med 2014;11(1): 222–9.

42. Elamin MB, Garcia MZ, Murad MH, et al. Effect of sex steroid use on cardiovascular risk in transsexual individuals: a systematic review and meta-analyses. Clin Endocrinol (Oxf) 2010;72(1):1–10.

43. Calof OM, Singh AB, Lee ML, et al. Adverse events associated with testosterone replacement in middle-aged and older men: a meta-analysis of randomized, placebo-controlled trials. J Gerontol 2005; 60(11):1451–7.

44. Giovanni C, Elisa M, Giulia R, et al. Cardiovascular risk associated with testosterone-boosting medications: a systematic review and meta-analysis. Expert Opin Drug Saf 2014;13(10):1327–51.

45. Van Caenegem E, Wierckx K, Taes Y, et al. Bone mass, bone geometry, and body composition in female-to-male transsexual persons after long-term cross-sex hormonal therapy. J Clin Endocrinol Metab 2012;97(7):2503–11.

46. Van Kesteren P, Lips P, Gooren LJG, et al. Long-term follow-up of bone mineral density and bone metabolism in transsexuals treated with cross-sex hormones. Clin Endocrinol (Oxf) 1998;48(3): 347–54.

47. Raigosa M, Avvedimento S, Yoon TS, et al. Male-to-female genital reassignment surgery: a retrospective review of surgical technique and complications in 60 patients. J Sex Med 2015;12(8):1837–45.

Preparing for Facial Feminization Surgery
Timing

Troy A. Pittman, MD[a],*, James M. Economides, MD[b]

KEYWORDS

- Transgender • Gender affirmation surgery • Facial feminization • Surgical timing

KEY POINTS

- Facial feminization surgery is part of a multifaceted treatment plan for gender dysphoria.
- Surgical intervention is often the last step in a process involving a mental health assessment, referral for hormonal treatment, and living in a gender-congruent role for at least 12 months.
- No guidelines exist specific to facial feminization surgery.
- The treating surgeon should use the Standards of Care for the Health of Transsexual, Transgender, and Gender Nonconforming People detailed by the World Professional Association of Transgender Health as a basis for the care of this patient population.

INTRODUCTION

The treatment of gender dysphoria is primarily composed of 3 separate, yet interrelated, modalities: (1) psychotherapy, (2) hormone therapy, and (3) surgical intervention. Early approaches historically focused primarily on sex reassignment surgeries to achieve a physical anatomic change from male to female or female to male, showing a remarkable increase in satisfaction rates of up to 87% in male-to-female (MTF) and 97% in female-to-male populations.[1–3] However, more recent investigations have demonstrated that hormone therapy combined with surgery may be necessary to alleviate gender dysphoria in a subset of patients.[4–6] Still, although many patients may require both hormone therapy and surgery to achieve symptomatic improvement, others may need only one or neither of these treatments.[7–9] The treatment of gender dysphoria and any consideration for surgical intervention must thus be made through interdisciplinary management involving a team of specialists from psychiatry, psychology, social work, endocrinology, gynecology, urology, and plastic surgery. Treatment guidelines are provided by the World Professional Association of Transgender Health (WPATH) and generally include (in this order) an initial mental health assessment, referral for hormonal therapy, and finally referral for surgical intervention (**Fig. 1**) with specific criteria for each step in the treatment process.

The World Professional Association of Transgender Health

The WPATH is an "international, multidisciplinary, professional association whose mission is to promote evidence-based care, education, research, advocacy, public policy, and respect for transgender health."[10] The WPATH outlines guidelines for the highest standards of health care for these individuals through the publication of the *Standards of Care (SOC) for the Health of Transsexual,*

Disclosures: The authors have no financial disclosures related to the preparation of this article.
[a] Advanced Plastic Surgery, 2440 M Street NW, Suite 507, Washington, DC 20037, USA; [b] Department of Plastic and Reconstructive Surgery, MedStar Georgetown University Hospital, Pasquerilla Health Center, 1st Floor, 3800 Reservoir Road Northwest, Washington, DC 20037, USA
* Corresponding author.
E-mail address: drpittman@pittmanmd.com

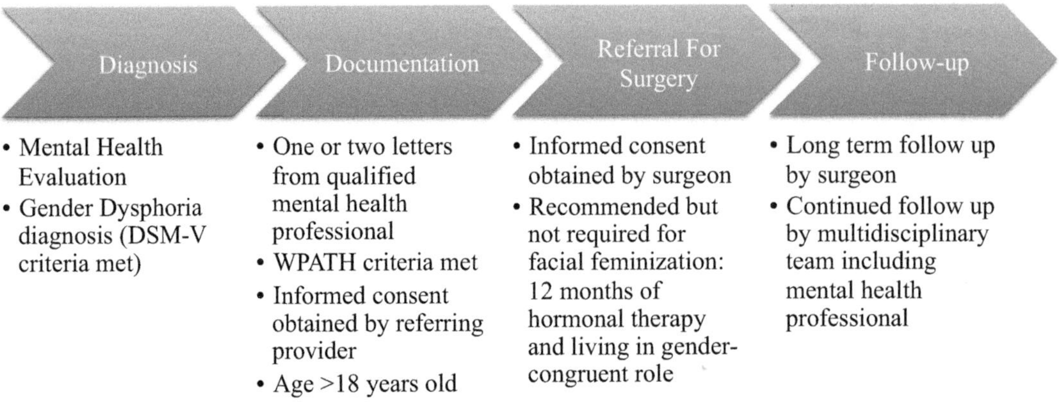

Fig. 1. Outline of a treatment plan for gender dysphoria. DSM-V, diagnostic and statistical manual of mental disorders, fifth edition; WPATH, world professional association of transgender health.

Transgender, and Gender Nonconforming People. The standard of care are the highest available science and expert consensus of the field with the goal to provide guidance for caretakers to assist the transsexual, transgender, and gender nonconforming populations achieve physical and mental well-being.

Initial Mental Health Assessment

The first step in the treatment of gender dysphoria is a mental health assessment by a trained professional. Mental health professionals who evaluate transgender patients should meet the basic requirements of the clinical competencies of their respective disciplines. These may include any discipline that prepares mental health professionals for clinical practice, including psychiatry, psychology, social work, mental health counseling, marriage and family therapy, nursing, or family medicine with additional training in behavioral health and counseling. The WPATH recommends the following minimum credentials for mental health professionals working with adults presenting with gender dysphoria[10]:

1. A master's degree or its equivalent in a clinical behavioral science field. This degree or a more advanced one should be granted by an institution accredited by the appropriate national or regional accrediting board. The mental health professional should have documented credentials from a relevant licensing board or equivalent for that country. Competence in using the *Diagnostic Statistical Manual of Mental Disorders* and/or the *International Classification of Diseases* for diagnostic purposes.
2. The ability to recognize and diagnose coexisting mental health concerns and to distinguish these from gender dysphoria.
3. Documented supervised training and competence in psychotherapy or counseling.
4. Knowledgeable about gender nonconforming identities and expressions, and the assessment and treatment of gender dysphoria.
5. Continuing education in the assessment and treatment of gender dysphoria. This training may include attending relevant professional meetings, workshops, or seminars; obtaining supervision from a mental health professional with relevant experience; or participating in research related to gender nonconformity and gender dysphoria.

The WPATH also recommends that in addition to these credentials, the mental health professional acquires and remains update on cultural competence with the transgender population to facilitate their treatment of these patients.

A diagnosis of gender dysphoria is made by meeting criteria as outlined in the *Diagnostic and Statistical Manual of Mental Disorders*, fifth edition, for children (**Box 1**) and adults (**Box 2**).[11] The mental health professional, through their ongoing assessment and work with the transgender patient will then make their recommendations and referrals for hormone therapy and/or surgery. They are also available to assist their patients considering surgery to be psychologically prepared for the endeavor; that is, that they have made a fully informed decision with clear and realistic postoperative expectations, have pursued surgery in line with the goals of their overall treatment plan, and have included family and/or friends as appropriate in their decision making.

Mental Health Referral For Hormone Therapy

Referrals for hormone therapy generally precede any surgical intervention and are made

Box 1
Diagnostic criteria for gender dysphoria in children

A. A marked incongruence between one's experienced/expressed gender and assigned gender, of at least 6 months' duration, as manifested by at least 6 of the following (one of which must be criterion A1):

   1. A strong desire to be of the other gender or an insistence that one is the other gender (or some alternative gender different from one's assigned gender).

   2. In boys (assigned gender), a strong preference for cross-dressing or simulating female attire; or in girls (assigned gender), a strong preference for wearing only typical masculine clothing and a strong resistance to the wearing of typical feminine clothing.

   3. A strong preference for cross-gender roles in make believe play or fantasy play.

   4. A strong preference for the toys, games, or activities stereotypically used or engaged in by the other gender.

   5. A strong preference for playmates of the other gender.

   6. In boys (assigned gender), a strong rejection of typically masculine toys, games, and activities and a strong avoidance of rough-and-tumble play; or in girls (assigned gender), a strong rejection of typically feminine toys, games, and activities.

   7. A strong dislike of one's sexual anatomy.

   8. A strong desire for the primary and/or secondary sex characteristics that match one's experienced gender.

B. The condition is associated with clinically significant distress or impairment in social, school, or other important areas of functioning.

Specify if:

• With a disorder of sex development (eg, a congenital adrenogenital disorder such as congenital adrenal hyperplasia or androgen insensitivity syndrome).

---

following a psychosocial assessment by a qualified health professional. The criteria for hormone therapy as outlined by the WPATH are as follows[10]:

1. Persistent, well-documented gender dysphoria.
2. Capacity to make a fully informed decision and to consent for treatment.
3. Age of majority in a given country.
4. If significant medical or mental health concerns are present, they must be reasonably well-controlled.

Feminizing hormone therapy induces physical changes that are more congruent with a patient's gender identity. Many of these changes occur over the course of up to 2 years and may be a permanent change. It is important to take these considerations into account when planning for any facial feminization procedure (**Table 1**).[12] In the MTF population, these effects include breast growth, decreased libido and erections, decreased testicular size, and increased body fat compared with muscle mass.

Mental Health Referral for Surgery

Surgery is often the final and most deliberated intervention in the treatment of gender dysphoria. Although many transgendered individuals may successfully find comfort in their gender identity, role, and expression without surgical intervention, many do find surgical intervention necessary to alleviate their symptoms of gender dysphoria.[13] Many studies have shown an improved sense of well-being, cosmesis, and sexual function after gender affirmation surgery.[14–17]

Surgical treatments for gender dysphoria require either 1 or 2 referrals from a qualified mental health professional, depending on the type of intervention. Currently, the WPATH Standards of Care do not specify criteria for procedures such as feminizing or masculinizing facial surgery; however, mental health professionals may play an important role in helping the patient to make an informed decision regarding the timing and importance of such procedures in their transition process. The mental health professional provides documentation of the patient's treatment history, progress, and overall eligibility. The WPATH has outlined the following

---

Box 2
Diagnostic criteria for gender dysphoria in adults

A. A marked incongruence between one's experienced/expressed gender and assigned gender, of at least 6 months' duration, as manifested by at least 2 of the following:

1. A marked incongruence between one's experienced/expressed gender and primary and/or secondary sex characteristics (or in young adolescents, the anticipated secondary sex characteristics).

2. A strong desire to be rid of one's primary and/or secondary sex characteristics because of a marked incongruence with one's experienced/expressed gender (or in young adolescents, a desire to prevent the development of the anticipated secondary sex characteristics).

3. A strong desire for the primary and/or secondary sex characteristics of the other gender.

4. A strong desire to be of the other gender (or some alternative gender different from one's assigned gender).

5. A strong desire to be treated as the other gender (or some alternative gender different from one's assigned gender).

6. A strong conviction that one has the typical feelings and reactions of the other gender (or some alternative gender different from one's assigned gender).

B. The condition is associated with clinically significant distress or impairment in social, occupational, or other important areas of functioning.

Specify if:

- With a disorder of sex development (eg, a congenital adrenogenital disorder such as congenital adrenal hyperplasia or androgen insensitivity syndrome).

- Coding note: Code the disorder of sex development as well as gender dysphoria.

Specify if:

- After transition: The individual has transitioned to full-time living in the desired gender (with or without legalization of gender change) and has undergone (or is preparing to have) at least 1 cross-sex medical procedure or treatment regimen—namely, regular cross-sex hormone treatment or gender reassignment surgery confirming the desired gender (eg, penectomy, vaginoplasty in a natal male; mastectomy or phalloplasty in a natal female).

Table 1
Effects and expected time course of feminizing hormones

Effect	Expected Onset	Expected Maximum Effect
Body fat redistribution	3–6 mo	2–5 y
Decreased muscle mass/strength	3–6 mo	1–2 y
Softening of skin/decreased oiliness	3–6 mo	Unknown
Decreased libido	1–3 mo	1–2 y
Decreased spontaneous erections	1–3 mo	3–6 mo
Male sexual dysfunction	Variable	Variable
Breast growth	3–6 mo	2–3 y
Decreased testicular volume	3–6 mo	2–3 y
Decreased sperm production	Variable	Variable
Thinning and slowed growth of body and facial hair	6–12 mo	>3 y
Male pattern baldness	No regrowth, loss stops 1–3 mo	1–2 y

Data from Hembree WC, Cohen-Kettenis P, Delemarre-van de Waal HA, et al. Endocrine treatment of transsexual persons: an Endocrine Society clinical practice guideline. J Clin Endocrinol Metab 2009;94(9):3132–54. Copyright 2009, The Endocrine Society.

recommendations for referral letters based on surgery type[10]:

1. One referral from a qualified mental health professional is needed for breast/chest surgery (eg, mastectomy, chest reconstruction, or augmentation mammoplasty).
2. Two referrals—from qualified mental health professionals who have independently assessed the patient—are needed for genital surgery (ie, hysterectomy/salpingo-oophorectomy, orchiectomy, and genital reconstructive surgeries). If the first referral is from the patient's psychotherapist, the second referral should be from a person who has only had an evaluative role with the patient.

The content of the referral letters for surgery should be the following:

1. The client's general identifying characteristics.
2. Results of the client's psychosocial assessment, including any diagnoses.
3. The duration of the mental health professional's relationship with the client, including the type of evaluation and therapy or counseling to date.
4. An explanation that the criteria for surgery have been met, and a brief description of the clinical rationale for supporting the patient's request for surgery.
5. A statement about the fact that informed consent has been obtained from the patient.
6. A statement that the mental health professional is available for coordination of care and welcomes a phone call to establish this.

Importantly, the WPATH maintains that the mental health professionals who recommend surgery share in the ethical and legal responsibilities for that decision with the surgeon. The WPATH outlines guidelines for the informed consent process, provided as an ethical and legal requirement for any surgical intervention.[10] These items include:

1. The different surgical techniques available (with referral to colleagues who provide alternative options).
2. The advantages and disadvantages of each technique.
3. The limitations of a procedure to achieve "ideal" results; surgeons should provide a full range of before-and-after photographs of their own patients, including both successful and unsuccessful outcomes.
4. The inherent risks and possible complications of the various techniques; surgeons should inform patients of their own complication rates with each procedure.

This information should be provided to the patient in writing and discussed in detail before proceeding. A minimum of 24 hours should be allowed for the patient to review this information privately and return with any questions for clarification.

Criteria for Surgery

Although no specific criteria exist for surgical feminization of the face, much may be gleaned from the criteria provided by the WPATH for other MTF surgical procedures. The WPATH criteria for nongenital surgery in MTF patients is as follows:

1. Persistent, well-documented gender dysphoria.
2. Capacity to make a fully informed decision and to consent for treatment.
3. Age of majority in a given country.
4. If significant medical or mental health concerns are present, they must be reasonably well-controlled.

It is worth noting that hormone therapy is not an explicit criterion to undergo nongenital (top) surgical intervention in either MTF or female-to-male transitions; however, it is generally recommended for a period of at least 12 months before surgery so that any feminizing effects may have achieved their maximum expected result. The WPATH does require at least 12 months of continuous hormone therapy for those patients undergoing gonadectomy and other genital surgery to allow for a period of reversible sex hormone suppression before undergoing irreversible surgical intervention.

The WPATH also does not require a period of living in an identity-congruent gender role for nongenital and gonadectomy surgeries. It does, however, require a period of at least 12 months of living in such a role for metoidoplasty/phalloplasty in female-to-male patients or vaginoplasty in MTF patients. The rationale behind this 12-month period is based on expert consensus that this period allows the patient ample opportunity to experience life in their desired gender role and adjust before undergoing an irreversible change. Transitioning to a new gender role has profound social consequences with many familial, interpersonal, vocational, education, social, economic, and legal challenges. Support from a mental health professional during this time is vital to ensuring a successful transition.[7] The duration of 12 months is important to allow the individual to experience the full range of different life experiences over the course of the year including holidays, vacations, seasons, and special events.

Postoperative Follow-up

Long-term postoperative follow-up after surgical treatment of gender dysphoria has been shown to be associated with good surgical and psychosocial outcomes.[18] Although postoperative patients often are lost to follow-up by specialty providers, these providers are generally the most apt to prevent, diagnose, or treat conditions to surgically treated patients. The need for follow-up with mental health professional postoperatively is also important as these professionals are well-suited to assisting in postoperative adjustment difficulties.

Insurance considerations

Considerations for the minor patient The phenomenology of gender dysphoria varies between children and adolescents primarily in the proportion of whom continue to experience symptoms through adulthood. Gender dysphoria during childhood is not guaranteed to persist through adulthood. In fact, studies have shown that, in prepubertal children referred for mental health assessment of gender dysphoria, symptoms persisted in 6% to 23% of male children and 12% to 27% in mixed gender cohorts.[19–21] In the adolescent population, the persistence of gender dysphoria into adulthood seems to be much greater. No prospective study exists to date; however, in a study of 70 adolescent patients who were diagnosed with gender dysphoria and treated with puberty suppressing hormones, 100% continued with sex reassignment therapy.[22]

Surgical intervention for transgender children and adolescents is generally not undertaken with many centers requiring patients to be over the age of majority. Physical interventions may be undertake for adolescents, however, and fall into 3 stages[12]:

1. Fully reversible interventions, including gonadotropin analogues to suppress sex hormones and delay the physical changes of puberty.
2. Partially reversible interventions including sex hormones whose effects may require reconstructive surgery to be reversed.
3. Irreversible interventions including surgical procedures.

The WPATH recommends a staged approach first, with fully reversible interventions, and then with partially reversible interventions to begin when pubertal changes commence. The decision to proceed in this manner is made by the patient and their parents and should also include close follow-up with a mental health professional as well as counseling for the patient's parents to engage in their child's transition. The WPATH recommends against genital surgery until the patient reaches the age of majority and they have lived continuously for 12 months in the gender role congruent with their gender identity. No guidelines exist for facial feminization surgery, however.[10]

SUMMARY

Facial feminization surgery may be a part of a multifaceted treatment plan for patients suffering from gender dysphoria. Initial assessment by a mental health professional must occur and referrals for hormonal therapy may then be made if deemed appropriate. Although no guidelines exist for timing of facial feminization surgery, it is generally recommended that individuals undergo hormonal therapy and live in a gender-congruent role for at least 12 months before surgical intervention. Additionally, letters of referral meeting WPATH guidelines must be made to outline the patient's treatment course and goals. Informed consent must be obtained with the patient understanding how surgical alteration of their appearance fits into their overall treatment goals.

REFERENCES

1. Benjamin H. The transsexual phenomenon. New York: Julian Press; 1966.
2. Green R, Fleming D. Transsexual surgery follow-up: status in the 1990s. Annu Rev Sex Res 1990;1(1): 163–74.
3. Hastings DW. Postsurgical adjustment of male transsexual patients. Clin Plast Surg 1974;1(2):335–44.
4. American Medical Association. Resolution 122 (A-08). 2008. Available at: http://www.ama-assn.org/ama1/pub/upload/mm/471/122.doc. Accessed June 20, 2018.
5. Anton BS. Proceedings of the American Psychological Association for the legislative year 2008: minutes of the annual meeting of the council of representatives, February 22-24, 2008, Washington, DC, and August 13 and 17, 2008, Boston, MA, and minutes of the February, June, August, and December 2008 meetings of the board of directors. Am Psychol 2009;64:372–453.
6. WPATH Board of Directors. Depsychopathologisation statement released May 26, 2010. 2010. Available at: http://wpath.org/announcements_detail.cfm?pk_announcement=17. Accessed June 20, 2018.
7. Bockting WO. Psychotherapy and the real-life experience: from gender dichotomy to gender diversity. Sexologies 2008;17(4):211–24.
8. Bockting WO, Goldberg JM. Guidelines for transgender care (special issue). Int J Transgend 2006; 9(3/4).

9. Lev AI. The ten tasks of the mental health provider: recommendations for revision of The World Professional Association for Transgender Health's standards of care. Int J Transgend 2009;11(2):74–99.

10. "Standards of care for the health of transsexual, transgender, and gender nonconforming People". The World Professional Association for Transgender Health. Version 7. Available at: www.wpath.org.

11. Gruenborg EM. Diagnostic and statistical manual of mental disorders 5. American Psychiatric Association; 2013. p. 459.

12. Hembree WC, Cohen-Kettenis P, Delemarre-van de Waal HA, et al. Endocrine treatment of transsexual persons: an Endocrine Society clinical practice guideline. J Clin Endocrinol Metab 2009;94(9):3132–54.

13. Hage JJ, Karim RB. Ought GIDNOS get nought? Treatment options for nontranssexual gender dysphoria. Plast Reconstr Surg 2000;105(3):1222–7.

14. De Cuypere G, T'Sjoen G, Beerten R, et al. Sexual and physical health after sex reassignment surgery. Arch Sex Behav 2005;34(6):679–90.

15. Gijs L, Brewaeys A. Surgical treatment of gender dysphoria in adults and adolescents: recent developments, effectiveness, and challenges. Annu Rev Sex Res 2007;18:178–224.

16. Klein C, Gorzalka BB. Sexual functioning in transsexuals following hormone therapy and genital surgery: a review (CME). J Sex Med 2009;6(11):2922–39.

17. Pfafflin F, Junge A. Sex reassignment. Thirty years of international follow-up studies after sex reassignment surgery: a comprehensive review, 1961-1991. Int J Transgend 1998. Available at: http://web.archive.org/web/20070503090247/http://www.symposion.com/ijt/pfaefflin/1000.htm. Accessed June 01, 2018.

18. Monstrey S, Hoebeke P, Selvaggi G, et al. Penile reconstruction: is the radial forearm flap really the standard technique? Plast Reconstr Surg 2009;124(2):510–8.

19. Cohen-Kettenis PT, Schagen SEE, Steensma TD, et al. Puberty suppression in a gender-dysphoric adolescent: a 22-year follow-up. Arch Sex Behav 2011;40(4):843–7.

20. Green R. The "sissy boy syndrome" and the development of homosexuality. New Haven (CT): Yale University Press; 1987.

21. Zucker KJ, Bradley SJ. Gender identity disorder and psychosexual problems in children and adolescents. New York: Guilford Press; 1995.

22. de Vries ALC, Steensma TD, Doreleijers TAH, et al. Puberty suppression in adolescents with gender identity disorder: a prospective follow-up study. J Sex Med 2010;8(8):2276–83. Advance online publication.

Cheek Augmentation Techniques

David M. Whitehead, MD, MS[a], Loren S. Schechter, MD, FACS[b],*

KEYWORDS

- Cheek augmentation • Midface • Facial feminization • FFS • Filler • Fat grafting • Facial implant
- Gender

KEY POINTS

- Sexual dimorphism of the lateral midface is primarily related to differences in the soft tissue rather than the underlying facial skeleton, and these soft tissue differences may be under hormonal control.
- Cheek augmentation can provide feminization by restoring youthful volume distribution within the aging midface.
- Surgical techniques can be directed at age-related changes in the facial skeleton, overlying soft tissue (eg, fat pads, fascia, skin), or both.
- Nonsurgical techniques can be used in isolation or in combination with surgical techniques.
- Caution should be exercised to avoid an "overfilled" appearance.

INTRODUCTION

Traditionally, gender-confirming procedures have focused on the breast and genitalia; however, the ability to socially transition may be most influenced by the face. Testosterone exposure leads to specific changes in the face within both the facial skeleton and overlying soft tissues. Facial feminization aims to reverse these changes, whether through surgical, nonsurgical (eg, injectables, skin-resurfacing), or nonmedical interventions (eg, cosmetics, hairpieces). Interventions include the goal of both reducing masculine features as well as providing a feminine appearance to the face. Distinct from feminizing procedures are those pertaining to rejuvenation. These interventions are aimed at reducing the effects of facial aging and may or may not be gender-specific.

The cheek encompasses the maxillary and zygomatic bones, as well as their overlying soft tissues, including the paranasal soft tissues. A feminine cheek is classically described as having higher and more prominent "cheekbones." Despite the use of the word "bones" in that term, it generally is used to refer to appearance of the soft tissues overlying the skeletal structures that make up the cheeks.

Several studies have sought to evaluate differences in the bony anatomy between male and female human faces (the terms male and female refer to individuals assigned to that sex at birth who subsequently underwent development into adulthood without the influence of exogenous hormones or an intersex state). An early cephalometric study demonstrated no significant difference in anterior bony malar projection between male and female participants,[1] represented by sella-nasion-orbitale (SNO) angle for the upper malar complex and pterygomaxillary vertical

Disclosures: Neither Dr D.M. Whitehead nor Dr L.S. Schechter (royalties from Elsevier publishing) have any financial conflicts of interest to declare.
[a] Division of Plastic Surgery, Department of Surgery, Northwell Health, 1991 Marcus Avenue, Suite 102, North New Hyde Park, NY 11042-2062, USA; [b] Private Practice, 9000 Waukegan Road, Suite 210, Morton Grove, IL 60053, USA
* Corresponding author.
E-mail address: lss@univplastics.com

Facial Plast Surg Clin N Am 27 (2019) 199–206
https://doi.org/10.1016/j.fsc.2018.12.003

to Key Ridge and Key Ridge to A point (PtV-KR/ KR-A) ratio for the lower malar complex. SNO angle was also shown to be similar between male and female individuals with a negative vector orbital relationship as compared with males and female individuals with a positive vector orbital relationship.[2] However, a more recent computed tomography study revealed subtle, but significant differences, between male and female zygoma that were conserved across ethnic groups.[3] Specifically, the female orbital rim had a slightly less acute curve, the body of the zygoma was slightly shorter in a vertical dimension, and the zygomatic arch demonstrated less bowing.

Conversely, the soft tissue differences appear to be more pronounced. Using soft tissue markers with cephalometric analysis in white patients, it was found that the soft tissue orbital rim, "cheek bone" (right malar greatest projection at three-fourths frontal view intersected by a vertical line through the lateral canthus on full frontal view), alar base (deepest depression of the alar rim), and subpupil (directly below the neutral gaze position of the pupil at one-half the vertical distance between the soft tissue orbital rim and the alar base marker) was significantly more projected in female than in male individuals. The converse was true in other areas of the face.[4] Similar findings were encountered in male and female individuals of Japanese descent.[5] With regard to a potential difference in cheek height, a photographic study found no significant difference in the height of greatest malar projection on oblique view relative to lateral canthus and chin, a value found to be slightly lower than the golden ratio of 0.809.[6] Due to a generally shorter lower face in female individuals, this may make the malar prominence appear closer to the eye or "higher," but the ratio showed no difference.

As suggested by Hage and colleagues,[7] the difference between the projection of the male and female midface appears to be primarily related to fat distribution. Missing from the current literature is an analysis of the facial volume changes brought on by the initiation of cross-sex hormones. Various online forums and personal accounts by transwomen describe a softening and rounding of their cheeks with estrogen treatment. This facial skin itself appears to change, with a decrease in sebum production, hair shaft diameter, and hair density. Similarly, for individuals designated female at birth undergoing testosterone treatment, there is a significant increase in hair growth and sebum production.[8] An increase in facial fat in the malar area, possibly as a result of feminizing hormones, may explain why this area is not frequently concerning to many younger transwomen seeking feminizing procedures.

An additional focus of the midface for any woman, trans- or cis-, appears to be age. Significant changes in both the soft tissue of the face and its underlying skeletal support occur over time, leading to an aged appearance (**Figs. 1–3**).

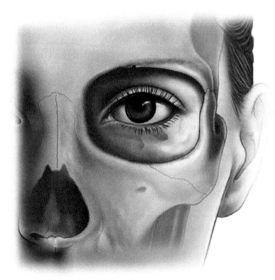 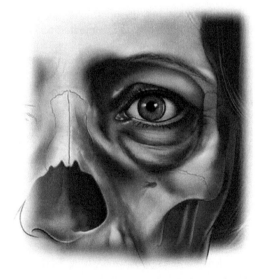

Fig. 1. Orbital and midfacial aging. This figure demonstrates a frontal view of the age-related changes in the facial skeleton. Note the bony resorption from the inferolateral orbit, pyriform aperture, and the maxilla overall. (*From* Mendelson B, Wong C-H. Changes in the facial skeleton with aging: implications and clinical applications in facial rejuvenation. Aesthetic Plast Surg 2012;36(4):754. Figure 1; with permission.)

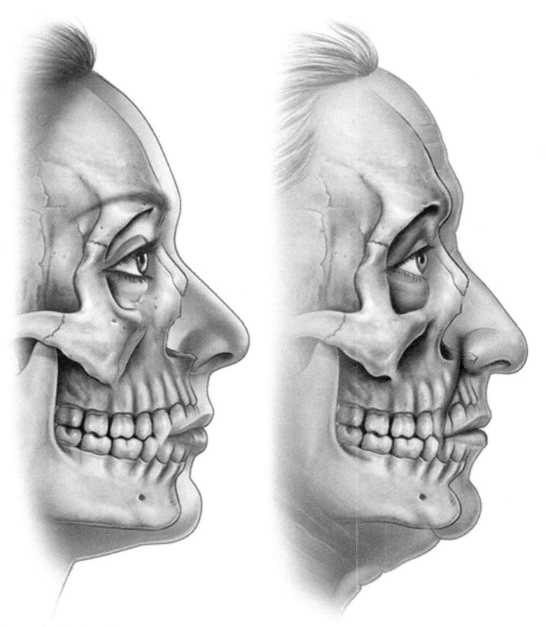

Fig. 2. Orbital and midfacial aging. This figure demonstrates a lateral view of the age-related changes in the facial skeleton. Note the bony resorption from the maxilla. (*From* Mendelson B, Wong C-H. Changes in the facial skeleton with aging: implications and clinical applications in facial rejuvenation. Aesthetic Plast Surg 2012;36(4):756. Figure 4; with permission.)

In the facial skeleton, there is significant retrusion of the maxilla over time, even in dentulous patients.[9–11] This includes significant widening of the pyriform aperture.[12] Resorption of the maxilla appears to be greatest at its ascending portion and at the lower pyriform. Although the zygoma appears less susceptible to age-related losses, there is still significant resorption at the inferolateral orbit. These skeletal changes lead to loss of bony midface support, accelerating descent of the soft tissues of the midface, accentuating the nasolabial folds, and causing recession of the anterior nasal spine, retraction of the columella, leading to ptosis of the nasal tip and the appearance of nasal lengthening.[13]

Meanwhile, through the forces of gravity, muscular activity, and loss of tissue elasticity, there is loss of projection of the malar soft tissues.

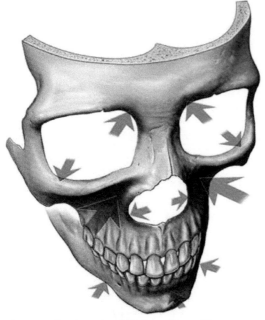

Fig. 3. Orbital and midfacial aging. Blue arrows demonstrate areas of bony resorption with advanced aging of the facial skeleton; larger arrows demonstrate areas of greater bone loss, clearly showing the maxilla as an area of significant resorption. (*From* Mendelson B, Wong C-H. Changes in the facial skeleton with aging: implications and clinical applications in facial rejuvenation. Aesthetic Plast Surg 2012;36(4):757. Figure 5; with permission.)

Descent of facial fat compartments (**Figs. 4** and **5**) (nasolabial, medial suborbicularis oculi, lateral suborbicularis oculi, medial cheek, and deep medial cheek), downward redistribution of volume and/or greatest sagittal diameter within the fat compartments (nasolabial and medial cheek), deflation and descent of the deep medial cheek fat compartment, as well as deflation of the buccal extension of the buccal fat pad have been documented.[14]

These 2 factors, skeletal and soft tissue, lend themselves to a variety of solutions. Although some obliquity to the malar eminence can be appealing,[15] overfilled cheeks or overprojected lateral zygomata can lead to an unnatural appearance. In fact, interzygomal distance is one of the least variable facial measurements within and between ethnic groups.[16]

TREATMENT OPTIONS
Injectable Dermal and Soft Tissue Fillers

Nonautologous fillers
A variety of commercially available dermal fillers have been used for augmentation of the midface. These include collagen-based fillers, volume replacement fillers such as hyaluronic acid, and biostimulatory fillers such as calcium hydroxyapatite and poly-L-lactic acid.[17]

The primary advantage of hyaluronic acid–based fillers is their temporary nature, as, over

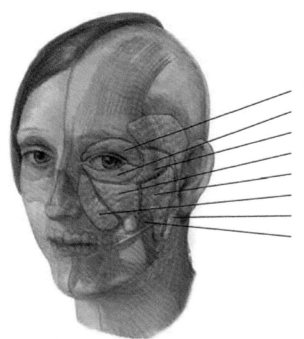

Superior orbital fat
Inferior orbital fat
Lateral orbital fat
Medial cheek fat
Middle cheek fat
Nasolabial fat
Lateral temporal-cheek fat
Buccal extension of the buccal fat

Fig. 4. Facial fat pads. Superficial fat pads of the face. (*From* Gierloff M, Stöhring C, Buder T, et al. Aging changes of the midfacial fat compartments: a computed tomographic study. Plast Reconstr Surg 2012;129(1):263. Figure 12; with permission)

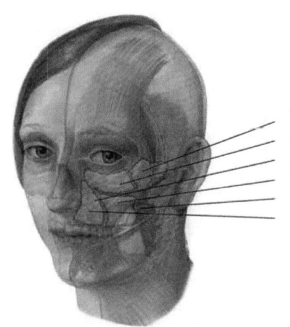

Sub—orbicularis oculi fat (lateral part)
Sub—orbicularis oculi fat (medial part)
Deep medial cheek fat (medial part)
Deep medial cheek fat (lateral part)
Buccal extension of the buccal fat
Ristow ´s space

Fig. 5. Facial fat pads. Deep fat pads of the face. (*From* Gierloff M, Stöhring C, Buder T, et al. Aging changes of the midfacial fat compartments: a computed tomographic study. Plast Reconstr Surg 2012;129(1):263. Figure 13; with permission.)

time, they will get degraded, the rate of which is inversely proportional to the amount of cross-linking in the filler. They also may be rapidly degraded by hyaluronidase in the event of complications. Hyaluronic acid fillers have been used to augment the zygomaticomalar area, antero-medial cheek, and submalar areas using both subcutaneous and supraperiosteal injection sites. They also have been used to efface the nasolabial fold and tear trough. Patients have reported that they looked younger after treatment, which persisted, in some, for up to 2 years.[18] Superficial injection of a significant amount of hyaluronic acid can lead to a bluish tint to the skin that some attribute to the Tyndall effect.[19] This can be addressed with the use of hyaluronidase.

Coralline calcium hydroxyapatite has been used to augment the facial skeleton over the anterior maxilla, zygoma, and mandibular body. In one study, a precise subperiosteal pocket was dissected out in the area to be augmented via a small access incision, and a mixture of the porous, granular calcium hydroxyapatite with blood and a hemostatic agent was introduced into the pocket, which was then closed. This demonstrated stable volume enhancement, and with time, also demonstrated bone ingrowth into the deep portion of filler material.[20]

Poly-L-lactic acid, which stimulates fibroblasts to produce collagen, has long been used to help combat the appearance of human immunodeficiency virus (HIV)-mediated lipodystrophy but has gained acceptance for use in non-HIV patients as well. It can be placed subcutaneously to efface skin creases like the nasolabial fold, or for greater volumization when placed along the periosteum.[21]

Autologous fat

Autologous fat, typically procured from the thighs or the anterior abdominal wall, is a frequently used soft tissue filler. It can be used to address volume deficits or contour problems in the nasolabial, nasojugal, malar, or submalar areas when injected in a subcutaneous or preperiosteal manner.[22]

More recently, attention has been directed to the facial fat compartments of the midface.[14] Use of direct fat injection into the deep medial fat compartment has been shown to efface the nasolabial fold and produce a more youthful appearance to the anterior cheek.[23] Others have demonstrated improved malar fullness when selectively injecting the medial and lateral suborbicularis oculi fat pads in addition to the deep medial fat pad.[24] Some have favored injection of the nasolabial, deep medial cheek, medial suborbicularis oculi, Ristow space, upper lip submucosa, and buccal extension of the buccal fat pad, for a satisfied or mostly satisfied rate of 95%.[25] There is also some evidence that direct injection into the buccal fat pad from an intraoral approach can effectively fill the midface.[26] The buccal fat pad has also been directly repositioned during LeFort I osteotomy to provide great fullness in the malar area.[27]

When injecting fat, it is expected that some resorption will likely occur. Traditional teaching suggests that 50% of the initial volume may be lost.[28,29] It is also taught that this figure can potentially be enhanced by grafting within highly vascular tissue, such as muscle. With less vascular tissue, it is unclear how predictable engraftment into the fat pads of the face may be, but some investigators demonstrate good, persistent results at 1 year.[25]

Potential complications of fillers

Caution should be used with fillers of any type, including fat. Intravascular filler injection in the midface can lead to soft tissue necrosis, blindness, and stroke. Intra-arterial filler injection can displace the blood and move as a pressure column up to the ciliary and retinal arteries, potentially leading to permanent blindness. If the column goes into the internal carotid artery, all structure that it supplies are at risk.[30] It is recommended that all injections be performed with a blunt cannula with, if possible, a sidefacing port.[23]

More common problems with injectable fillers include overfilling or underfilling, filling at an inappropriate tissue depth, filling at an inappropriate or suboptimal location, use of an inappropriate filler, as well as infectious or allergic complications. Many complications, if involving a hyaluronic acid–based filler, can be addressed, at least in part, with hyaluronidase. For other fillers, other strategies must be used.[31]

IMPLANTS

Given the skeletal contribution of loss of midface projection with age, some practitioners choose to use implants to augment the midfacial skeleton (**Fig. 6**), especially in individuals with negative vector orbital relationship for whom it can be said that

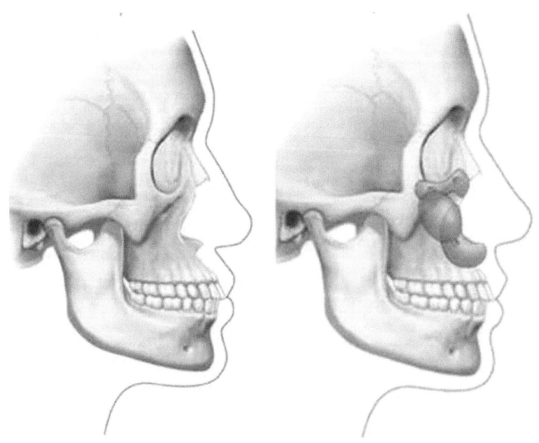

Fig. 6. Facial implants. This figure demonstrates a potential configuration of midface implants to enhance fullness of the cheek, including inferior orbital rim, malar eminence, and paranasal placement. (*Adapted from* Yaremchuk MJ. Making concave faces convex. Aesthetic Plast Surg 2005;29(3):142. Figure 1C and 1D; with permission.)

the descent of midfacial structures with age is accelerated.

The 2 most common implant types are silicone and porous polyethylene. Defenders of solid silicone facial implants suggest there are many advantages to this type implant. These include customizability through simple cutting of the implant with a scissor or a blade, easy removal, and potential for placement through a smaller access incision due to the flexibility of the material.[32] Those who prefer porous polyethylene implants favor their permanence through soft tissue integration (with decreased encapsulation), as well as their customizability both at the time of placement, and in the future, with the use of a burr.[33]

The infraorbital region may be addressed with an implant. An implant can help attenuate the tear trough, provide greater support to the lower lid and midface soft tissues, and potentially produce a positive vector relationship.[34] In addition, the anterolateral maxilla, lateral to the infraorbital foramen, also may be addressed with an implant. Here, the implant can help support the midmalar tissues, fill out the nasolabial fold, and reduce the prominence of the nose.[35,36] Implant placement also can be combined with soft tissue suspension to improve malar fullness.[33]

However, all types of facial implants can become infected and/or extrude. In addition, they can be associated with hematoma and/or persistent swelling. Encapsulation of the implants can lead to distortion of the overlying soft tissues. Furthermore, malpositioning is a possibility that can occur despite screw fixation. Many of these complications require subsequent removal of the implant, and all are important to discuss at the time of consultation and during the informed consent process.[37]

OTHER TECHNIQUES

Rhytidectomy to address skin excess can be a useful adjunct to the previously described techniques, likely as part of a staged approach.

In addition, some have suggested using an osteotomy with advancement of the zygomaticomalar complex, based on that of the LeFort III, for facial feminization.[38]

SUMMARY

The primary goal of midface procedures is feminization through volume augmentation. Additional, secondary benefits may include a rejuvenated appearance. Careful analysis of an individual's midface soft tissue structure and skeletal relationship can help dictate the treatment offered. Some individuals may benefit from injectable fillers or autologous fat grafting, whereas others may require a staged approach, using implant placement, fat grafting, and rhytidectomy.

REFERENCES

1. Scheideman GB, Bell WH, Legan HL, et al. Cephalometric analysis of dentofacial normals. Am J Orthod 1980;78(4):404–20.
2. Frey ST. New diagnostic tenet of the esthetic midface for clinical assessment of anterior malar projection. Angle Orthodontist 2013;83(5):790–4.
3. Schlager S, Rüdell A. Sexual dimorphism and population affinity in the human zygomatic structure—comparing surface to outline data. Anat Rec (Hoboken) 2017;300(1):226–37.
4. Arnett GW, Jelic JS, Kim J, et al. Soft tissue cephalometric analysis: diagnosis and treatment planning of dentofacial deformity. Am J Orthod Dentofacial Orthop 1999;116(3):239–53.
5. Shindoi JM, Matsumoto Y, Sato Y, et al. Soft tissue cephalometric norms for orthognathic and cosmetic surgery. J Oral Maxillofac Surg 2013;71(1):e24–30.
6. Kaptein YE, Kaptein JS, Markarian A. Vertical localization of the malar prominence. Plast Reconstr Surg Glob Open 2015;3(6). https://doi.org/10.1097/GOX.0000000000000383.
7. Hage JJ, Becking AG, de Graaf FH, et al. Gender-confirming facial surgery: considerations on the masculinity and femininity of faces. Plast Reconstr Surg 1997;99(7):1799.
8. Giltay EJ, Gooren LJG. Effects of sex steroid deprivation/administration on hair growth and skin sebum production in transsexual males and females. J Clin Endocrinol Metab 2000;85(8):2913–21.
9. Pessa JE, Zadoo VP, Mutimer KL, et al. Relative maxillary retrusion as a natural consequence of aging: combining skeletal and soft-tissue changes into an integrated model of midfacial aging. Plast Reconstr Surg 1998;102(1):205.
10. Mendelson BC, Hartley W, Scott M, et al. Age-related changes of the orbit and midcheek and the implications for facial rejuvenation. Aesthetic Plast Surg 2007;31(5):419–23.
11. Paskhover B, Durand D, Kamen E, et al. Patterns of change in facial skeletal aging. JAMA Facial Plast Surg 2017;19(5):413–7.
12. Shaw RBJ, Kahn DM. Aging of the midface bony elements: a three-dimensional computed tomographic study. Plast Reconstr Surg 2007;119(2):675.
13. Mendelson B, Wong C-H. Changes in the facial skeleton with aging: implications and clinical applications in facial rejuvenation. Aesthetic Plast Surg 2012;36(4):753–60.

14. Gierloff M, Stöhring C, Buder T, et al. Aging changes of the midfacial fat compartments: a computed tomographic study. Plast Reconstr Surg 2012; 129(1):263.

15. Paul MD. Morphologic and gender considerations in midface rejuvenation. Aesthet Surg J 2001;21(4): 349–53.

16. Fang F, Clapham PJ, Chung KC. A systematic review of inter-ethnic variability in facial dimensions. Plast Reconstr Surg 2011;127(2):874–81.

17. Lorenc ZP. Dermal and soft-tissue fillers: principles, materials, and techniques. In: Thorne CH, editor. Grabb and Smith's plastic surgery. 7th edition. Philadelphia: Lippincott Williams & Wilkins; 2014.

18. Few J, Cox SE, Paradkar-Mitragotri D, et al. A multicenter, single-blind randomized, controlled study of a volumizing hyaluronic acid filler for midface volume deficit: patient-reported outcomes at 2 years. Aesthet Surg J 2015;35(5):589–99.

19. Rootman DB, Lin JL, Goldberg R. Does the Tyndall effect describe the blue hue periodically observed in subdermal hyaluronic acid gel placement? Ophthalmic Plast Reconstr Surg 2014;30(6):524–7.

20. Huggins RJ, Mendelson BC. Biologic behavior of hydroxyapatite used in facial augmentation. Aesthetic Plast Surg 2017;41(1):179–84.

21. Rotunda AM, Narins RS. Poly-L-lactic acid: a new dimension in soft tissue augmentation. Dermatol Ther 2006;19(3):151–8.

22. Gamboa GM, Ross WA. Autologous fat transfer in aesthetic facial recontouring. Ann Plast Surg 2013; 70(5):513–6.

23. Rohrich RJ, Pessa JE, Ristow B. The youthful cheek and the deep medial fat compartment. Plast Reconstr Surg 2008;121(6):2107.

24. Schreiber JE, Terner J, Stern CS, et al. The boomerang lift: a three-step compartment-based approach to the youthful cheek. Plast Reconstr Surg 2018;141(4):910.

25. Wang W, Xie Y, Huang R-L, et al. Facial contouring by targeted restoration of facial fat compartment volume: the midface. Plast Reconstr Surg 2017; 139(3):563.

26. Cohen SR, Fireman E, Hewett S, et al. Buccal fat pad augmentation for facial rejuvenation. Plast Reconstr Surg 2017;139(6):1273e.

27. Hernández-Alfaro F, Valls-Ontañón A, Blasco-Palacio JC, et al. Malar augmentation with pedicled buccal fat pad in orthognathic surgery: three-dimensional evaluation. Plast Reconstr Surg 2015; 136(5):1063.

28. Peer LA. Loss of weight AND volume in human fat grafts: with postulation of A "cell survival theory." Plast Reconstr Surg 1950;5(3):217.

29. Bellini E, Grieco MP, Raposio E. The science behind autologous fat grafting. Ann Med Surg (Lond) 2017; 24:65–73.

30. Yoshimura K, Coleman SR. Complications of fat grafting: how they occur and how to find, avoid, and treat them. Clin Plast Surg 2015;42(3):383–8.

31. DeLorenzi C. Complications of injectable fillers, part I. Aesthet Surg J 2013;33(4):561–75.

32. Niamtu J. Essentials of cheek and midface implants. J Oral Maxillofac Surg 2010;68(6):1420–9.

33. Yaremchuk MJ. Making concave faces convex. Aesthetic Plast Surg 2005;29(3):141–7.

34. Yaremchuk MJ, Kahn DM. Periorbital skeletal augmentation to improve blepharoplasty and midfacial results. Plast Reconstr Surg 2009;124(6):2151.

35. Yaremchuk MJ, Vibhakar D. Pyriform aperture augmentation as an adjunct to rhinoplasty. Clin Plast Surg 2016;43(1):187–93.

36. Chao JW, Lee JC, Chang MM, et al. Alloplastic augmentation of the Asian face: a review of 215 patients. Aesthet Surg J 2016;36(8):861–8.

37. Rayess HM, Svider P, Hanba C, et al. Adverse events in facial implant surgery and associated malpractice litigation. JAMA Facial Plast Surg 2018;20(3):244–8.

38. Lundgren TK, Farnebo F. Midface osteotomies for feminization of the facial skeleton. Plast Reconstr Surg Glob Open 2017;5(1):e1210.

Forehead and Orbital Rim Remodeling

Marcelo Di Maggio, MD

KEYWORDS

- Forehead and orbital rim remodeling • Facial feminization surgery
- Facial features remodeling surgery • Frontal sinus reconstruction • Eye expression
- Periorbital aesthetic surgery • Craniofacial surgery • Aesthetic craniofacial surgery

KEY POINTS

- The concepts of forehead and orbital rim remodeling are explained and defined within the facial features remodeling surgery.
- The author gives the details of the surgical technique and indication at the forehead and orbital remodeling during the facial feminization surgery.
- The author describes different osteotomies used to address the forehead, orbital rim, and frontal sinus and the technique evolution over time.
- The author defines the aesthetic orbital, periorbital, and craniofacial surgery to modify the expression of the eyes and reports the aesthetic outcomes achieved with this approach.

INTRODUCTION

In recent years, there has been a growing appreciation of the negative psychosocial impact of facial feature dysphoria and gender dysphoria (GD) on quality of life, especially in the transgender community. With growing acceptance that treatment is warranted, more patients are seeking complete modification of their facial features that only craniofacial techniques can achieve.[1]

The author uses the term, *facial features remodeling surgery* (FFRS), for patients undergoing surgery to change their overall facial features, regardless of their gender or motivation. FFRS includes the concepts of forehead and orbital rim remodeling and facial feminization surgery (FFS) as well as additional craniofacial and aesthetic procedures to treat and remodel the entirety of the face by simultaneously addressing the soft tissue changes associated with aging as well as correcting any disharmony in the facial bony framework. The most dramatic changes can be achieved in only 1 or 2 procedures, with 10 days between one and the other. The treatment of the forehead and orbital rim remodeling is done along with the rest of the aesthetic and craniofacial procedures included in the FFRS. Those dramatic changes have been most evident in the author's patients with GD who want to transition from male to female appearance but have also been applicable to patients who have facial feature dysphoria unrelated to GD. The author's approach includes some new techniques to address the fronto-orbital region to obtain more effective feminization of the face.

FFRS represents the current stage in the evolution of the author's approach to FFS. To optimize the results of gender reassignment surgeries, it is necessary to have a multidisciplinary approach and to create an integrated program with emphasis on continuous learning, hopefully with institutional support (**Fig. 1**).

Disclosure statement: The author has nothing to disclose.
MDM Surgery Center, Sanatorio Finochietto Medical Center, Buenos Aires, Avenida Cordoba 2678, C1187AAN, Argentina
E-mail address: dimaggiomarcelo@gmail.com

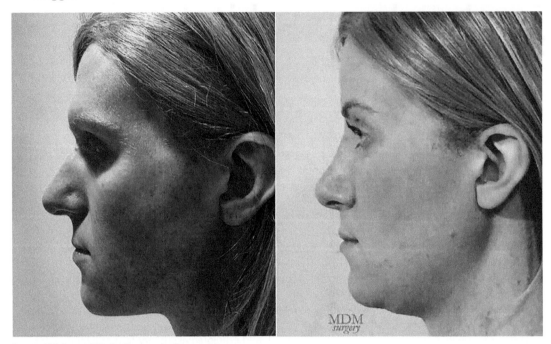

Fig. 1. FFRS and FFS, before and after results.

FRONTO-ORBITAL AESTHETICS AND FACIAL FEMINIZATION

The concepts of beauty and facial rejuvenation have been studied and documented since the beginnings of plastic surgery.[2] There is a close relationship between female beauty and the femininity of facial features. Masculine features detract from this aesthetic ideal. Anatomic differences between female and male skulls have been evaluated and show extreme divergence in the forehead, orbital rim, and jaw regions.[3,4] In men, the forehead is flat, with prominent supraorbital ridges. The female forehead is vertically higher and more rounded, with a smoother gentle arc. In relative proportions of the overall facial mass, the orbits in women are larger and appear higher. The male eyebrows are heavier, straighter, and closer to the eyes. In contrast, a woman's eyebrows are more arched. The soft, delicate, and sincere female expression can be attributed partly to this wider opening of the orbits. Female orbital margins are sharper and rounded.[5,6] The concept of FFS was initially reported by Ousterhout in 1987,[4] by stating which patterns to be considered to remodel a face and by introducing the first osteotomies for this purpose. Although the author still uses many of these concepts and techniques, the approach and incorporated complementary procedures have been modified in an attempt to achieve a comprehensive improvement in a shorter time course (**Fig. 2**).

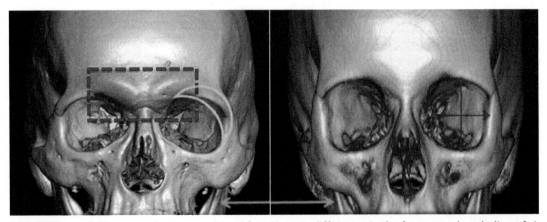

Fig. 2. Different skull anatomy between male and female. Main differences in the fronto-nasal angle (*in red*), in the superior orbital rim (*in yellow*).

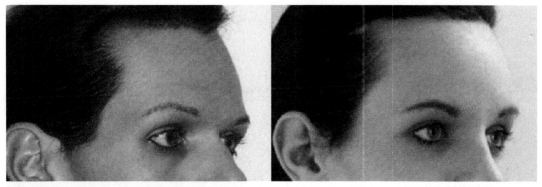

Fig. 3. Change in the eyes' expression after forehead and orbital remodeling. Before and after results.

The change in the eyes' expression is an important achievement with his surgical technique. This point is one of the strengths of the results and a main one when considering FFRS. What eyes can express goes beyond words and is the beginning of any social interaction. The author believes this improvement is an important change in comparison with other techniques that describe facial features remodeling. Including the frontonasal angle and the upper part of the nasal bone allowed designing and sculpting naturally and with harmony this fundamental transition zone when remodeling the upper third of the face[7,8] (**Fig. 3**).

There was a learning stage in the evolution of FFS techniques and the author has developed what is now called FFRS, which has its main basis in the treatment of the upper third of the face, the remodeling of the bone flap, and the frontal sinus. The anatomy of the frontal sinus is the main parameter to be taken into account, among other criteria (**Table 1**). As discussed previously, manipulating the frontal sinus ensures that the front flap can be reset in any type of reconstruction of the forehead or orbital rim. The remodeling of the frontal flap, its reset, and implant inside the sinus has improved the aesthetic results. The aforementioned procedures and the orbital remodeling and frontonasal angle allow a bigger set back, which can be seen in the quality of the results[9–15] (**Box 1**).

DESCRIPTION OF THE NEW FOREHEAD AND ORBITAL RIM OSTEOTOMIES AND REMODELING

Following the criteria for inclusion under forehead and orbital rim remodeling explained in the **Box 1**, the design of the osteotomies is planned before surgery by considering the aesthetic

Table 1
Facial features remodeling surgery

A—One-Stage Surgery Complete Facial Features Bone Remodeling	B—Two-Stage Surgery Complete Facial Features Bone Remodeling Plus Facial Soft Tissue Remodeling
1. Forehead and orbital rim remodeling (frontal sinus, supraorbital rim, and orbital aperture)	First step
	1. Jaw remodeling (angles, ramus, and chin)
2. Jaw remodeling (angles, ramus, and chin)	2. Face and neck lifting
3. Rhinoplasty (frontonasal region and tip angle)	3. Midface soft tissue pexy, cheek prosthesis, and/or fat transfer
4. Eyebrow lifting and hairline treatment	4. Upper lip lifting
5. Midface soft tissue pexy, cheek prosthesis, and/or fat transfer	5. Adam's apple (thyroid cartilage) contouring
6. Blepharoplasty, canthoplasty, and canthopexy	6. Orthognathic surgery
7. Upper lip lifting	Second step
8. Adam's apple (thyroid cartilage) treatment	1. Forehead and orbital rim remodeling (frontal sinus, supraorbital rim, and top and lateral and midwalls)
9. Hair implants	2. Rhinoplasty (frontal-nasal region and tip angle)
	3. Eyebrow lifting and hairline treatment
	4. Blepharoplasty, canthoplasty, and canthopexy
	5. Hair implant
	6. Others

Box 1
The criteria for inclusion under forehead and orbital rim remodeling—indications

1. FFS

2. Overdeveloped or protruding frontal sinus

3. Sharp frontonasal angle

4. Prominent frontal and orbital structures

5. Surgery to change the eyes expression (too strong, sad, or aged)

6. Orbital or periorbital aging

7. Classic facial aesthetic and rejuvenation treatment

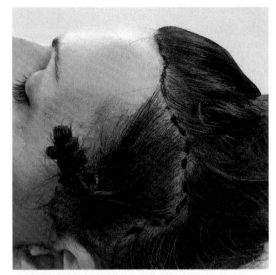

Fig. 5. Forehead incision. Medial hairline and lateral intrahairline design.

requirements and the anatomic characteristics of the frontal region.

The approach is via a bicoronal incision, either pretrichial or trichial, and other variations of incisions, depending on the need to change the shape of the hairline contour or the need to lower the hairline. Subgaleal dissection proceeds to 1 cm above the cephalic limit of the frontal sinus; then the periosteum is opened and subperiosteal dissection is performed to expose the fronto-orbital-nasal region (frontal sinus, supraorbital and lateral orbital rim, orbital roof and walls, frontonasal suture, and nasal dorsum), in all cases preserving and releasing the supraorbital and supratrochlear neurovascular structures and preserving the facial nerve branches (**Figs. 4** and **5**).

The cephalic limits of the frontal osteotomy coincide with the beginning of the protrusion of the anterior wall of the frontal sinus. The lateral limits vary but most commonly approximate an imaginary vertical line at the level of the supraorbital notch. Lateral extensions are made following the upper orbital rim. The lower limit goes as far as 1 cm below the frontonasal suture and to the border of the orbits. The osteotomy is performed after exposing the entire surface of the frontal sinus. Ostectomy of the bony projection of the superolateral rim is performed to reduce the anterior projection in this region along with contouring of the superior border of the orbit to increase the orbital height with the aim of converting the shape of the male orbital aperture into a more feminine configuration.

Treatment of the frontal sinus varies according to its anatomy, taking into consideration the size, depth, extension, and ostium type[16–18] (**Figs. 6** and **7**).

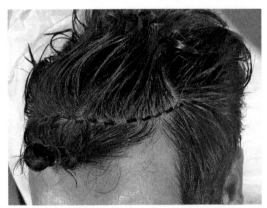

Fig. 4. Forehead incision. Medial intrahairline and lateral hairline design.

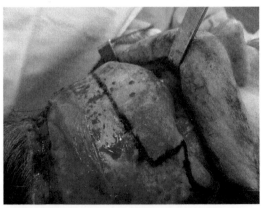

Fig. 6. Author's forehead and orbital rim osteotomy, design 1.

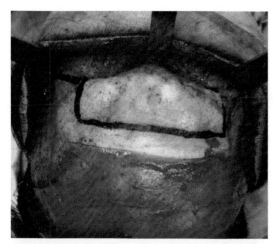

Fig. 7. Author's forehead and orbital rim osteotomy, design 2.

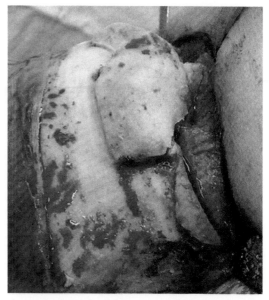

Fig. 8. Author's forehead and orbital rim osteotomy and remodeling.

In most cases, the frontal sinus mucosa is removed for technical reasons because the remodeled frontal bone flap is placed inside the sinus, leaving it smaller and completely permeable.

Next the anterior frontal bone flap is remodeled, configuring the shape, size, and projection to recess it within the frontal sinus, fixing bone edges with precision to avoid osteosynthesis materials, except in certain instances where small-caliber wire is used or, as an exception, titanium mesh to augment stability. The contouring is finished using bone chips and bone paste to cover minimum details. Finally, before finishing with the fronto-orbital remodeling, the frontonasal bridge and the nasal dorsum are remodeled, generally involving a ostectomy of approximately 1 cm when necessary. This is done to achieve a natural frontonasal angle that is coherent with the rhinoplasty also done when finishing the remodeling of the forehead and orbits.

Throughout the surgical procedure, a suction strainer is used to collect bone dust and all bone fragments are retained for use during the contouring of the frontal region. Finally, the periosteal flap is reset and the tissues closed in layers. If hairline remodeling or lateral eyebrow lifting is necessary, it is performed at this time. It is important to clarify that the reposition of the forehead flap bone inside the frontal sinus, along with the treatment of the nasal dorsum and the complete remodeling of the orbit, entails the objective of achieving the best possible aesthetic result, with a larger setback of the frontal and orbital region, a more feminine frontonasal angle, and a more noticeable change in the expression of the eyes. In general, other surgeons reposition the frontal flap bone at the same level as the rest of the forehead bone; therefore, they do not remove the mucosa of the frontal sinus and use microtitanium plates to fix it in place. There is an option of doing the regular rhinoplasty with the classic approach and also choosing to be less aggressive with the orbital remodeling. Everything depends on the result that the patient and surgeon are looking for.[19–23]

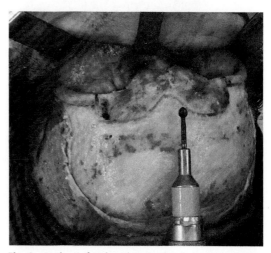

Fig. 9. Author's forehead and orbital rim remodeling.

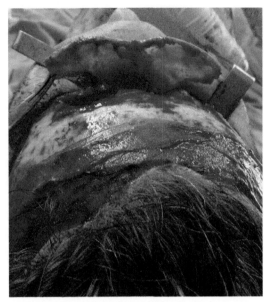

Fig. 10. Author's frontal and orbital osteotomy 1.

Usually the forehead and orbital rim remodeling that the author does in most patients includes rhinoplasty and frontal and eyebrow lift, along with blepharoplasty, hairline lowering, and shape correction when necessary (**Figs. 8–10**).

Regarding the hairline remodeling, the author tries to lower it as much as possible but without compromising the blood flow or increasing the tension that later translates into a bad and wide scar, hypertrophy or even dehiscence, and possible infection. Priority is given performing the frontal and orbital reconstruction without

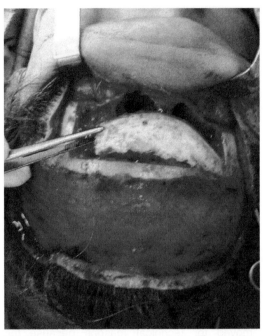

Fig. 12. Author's frontal osteotomy and frontal sinus remodeling.

complications. Logically, the author tries to modify the usual M-shape male pattern for a feminine one (**Fig. 11**).

What the patient expects and the possibilities of success of the option chosen are taken into consideration. A hairline incision can be done if advancing and lowering the hairline are desired, closing the usual lateral entrances and at the same time performing a better eyebrow lift.

The author chooses the classic bicoronal incision if a patient requests it or if it is not necessary to advance and lower the hairline. The eyebrows' reposition is always kept in mind in discussion with patients.

Sometimes, a combination of internal and external hairline incision is performed; in general,

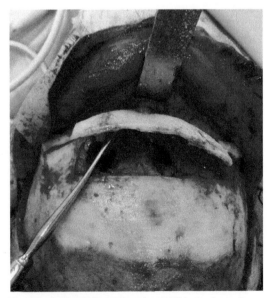

Fig. 11. Author's frontal and orbital osteotomy 2.

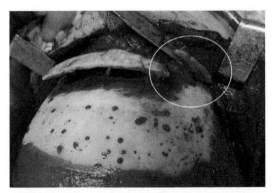

Fig. 13. Author's frontal and orbital rim osteotomy. Detail of the superior and lateral orbital osteotomy.

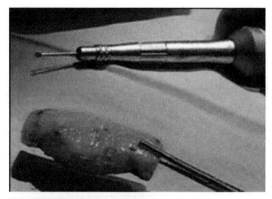

Fig. 14. Frontal bone remodeling.

it is done in patients who do not need to advance the frontal midline of the scalp but need to improve the shape and closing of the lateral entrances. With this option, the midarea incision is taken 2 cm or 3 cm behind the hairline and then the external incision continued at the beginning of the lateral entrance; so after the entrance is finished, it becomes an internal hairline incision again that is placed at the level of the temporal bone (the latter is the usual pattern in all the author's incisions, so after the lateral entrances are finished, the incision is always continued and it is finished within the hairline) (**Fig. 12**).

The usual average advance is 1.5 cm to 2 cm in the best circumstances. This advance could be lower if there is a greater dissection of the scalp reaching the occipital region, but the author prefers to be cautious in this point, always taking care of the frontal and orbital reconstruction and the quality of the final scar, which are very important.

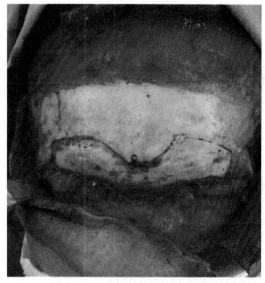

Fig. 16. Frontal bone flap placed into the frontal sinus and fixed with a small wire.

The author prefers to not use alloplastic materials to fix the scalp (to make up for the hairline lowering and the eyebrow lift) at this stage because of trying to avoid seromas and other complications.

In relation to the eyebrow lift, the author prioritizes repositioning the eyebrows in a natural way, which usually go up some millimeters after the posterior and vertical dissection and remodeling of the orbits. In these cases, a classic bicoronal incision is used; later, an anterior lateral incision to rise the eyebrows can be used.

In some patients, it is necessary to compensate the temporal regions and, in such cases, a porous polyethylene prosthesis or fat transfer or fillers are used.

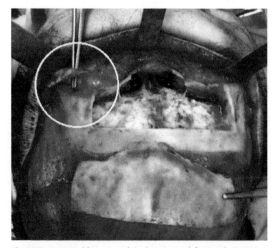

Fig. 15. Frontal bone, orbital rim, and frontal sinus remodeling. Detail of the superior and lateral orbital osteotomy.

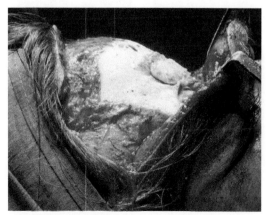

Fig. 17. Frontal bone reposition. Lateral view of the forehead remodeling.

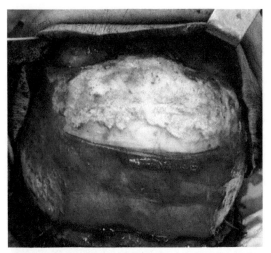

Fig. 18. Forehead and orbital rim remodeling after finishing touches made with bone chips and bone paste to achieve a smooth result.

The hair implant is strongly recommended to hide scars, to complete the hairline lowering, or to solve lateral entrances. In some cases, when the number of implants is small, they are done along with the frontal and orbital remodeling surgery and, in other cases, when the number of implants is bigger, the author prefers to do it at least 7 days to 10 days after the FFRS in another ambulatory surgery with local anesthesia or even later according to patient preference. The author believes that doing the hair implants as a separate procedure from the frontal surgery allows the FFS

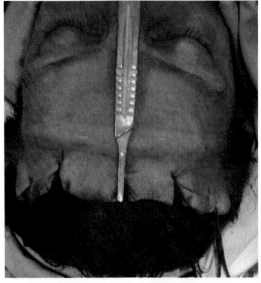

Fig. 19. Hairline lowering after the forehead remodeling.

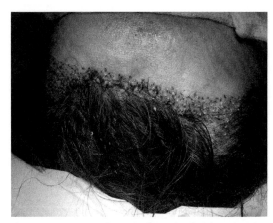

Fig. 20. Hair transplants before the hairline incision and in the lateral receding hairline to make the shape of the hairline more feminine.

to have a better postsurgery situation with less edema and complication risks as well as a better result. The advantage of performing it in the same frontal surgery is that hair from the scalp that is usually dismissed can be used[24–27] (**Figs. 13–20**).

RESULTS

The author considers the remodeling of the fronto-orbital region the most important aspect of FFRS, and it is one of the only procedures performed in all patients. This procedure (forehead and orbital rim remodeling) takes 120 minutes on average. Patients are hospitalized in an ordinary individual room and no intensive care unit monitoring was required for any of the cases. Patients left the hospital 24 hours after the surgery and in all cases the drains were removed before they were discharged.

The author found improvement in the results obtained, achieving a high level of satisfaction in the patients; combining bony and soft tissue procedures led to a better outcome due to the subperiosteal detachment performed before the osteotomies, and bone remodeling provided excellent mobilization for a possible lifting or any other soft tissue repositioning procedure that is wanted.

Intraoperative complications are not usual and they are in direct relation to the expertise of the medical team. Postoperative complications occur in approximately 5% of patients; infection in the forehead and frontal sinus, late mucoceles, hematomas and 1 hemorrhage, subcutaneous seromas, paresis of the frontal branch of the facial nerve, nonpermanent loss of the sensitivity of the forehead, infections due to alloplastic or titanium

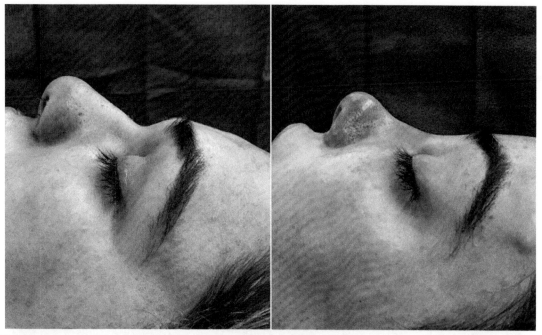

Fig. 21. Before and after right after the surgery. Forehead, orbital rim, and rhinoplasty results. Lateral view to see the difference in the frontonasal angle. Before and after results.

materials, partial dehiscence, and hypertrophic scarring are the most frequent.[18,28]

TECHNIQUE EVOLUTION IN RELATION TO THE TREATMENT OF THE FRONTAL SINUS

The author's original approach to the fronto-orbital region was similar to Ousterhout's[4,22,26,27] and most other FFS surgeons', in that a frontal osteotomy was performed and the bone flap remodeled and then replaced using titanium miniplates for fixation. There was no manipulation of the frontal sinus mucosa and a small shave at the supraorbital rim. At the same time, there was the option of the defunctionalization of the sinus in a small percentage of patients when considered convenient. The mucosa was burred out and the cavity treated with bone chips and bone paste to

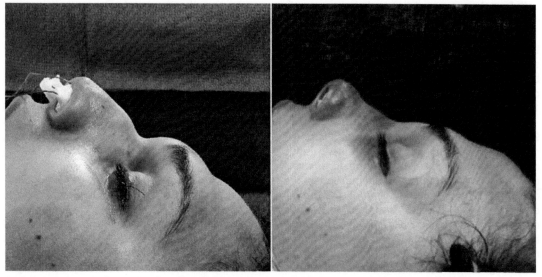

Fig. 22. Before and after right after the surgery. Forehead, orbital rim, and rhinoplasty results. Before and after results.

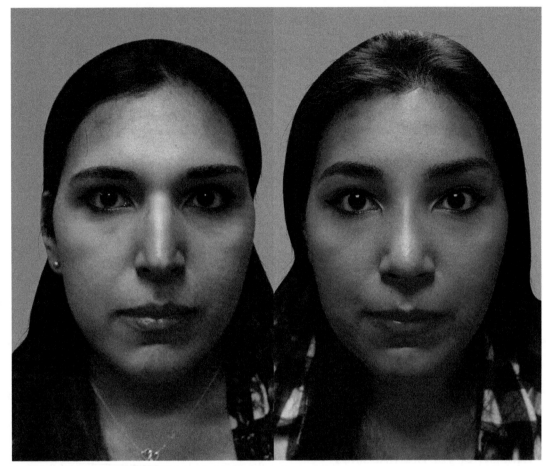

Fig. 23. Before and after results, patient 1. Before and after results.

block the sinus and then the frontal bone plate resecured with titanium plates and screws. With both frontal sinus remodeling techniques, complications were described (infection and mucocele). The author's current approach now involves selective sinus ablation with avoidance of plates and screws and special attention to reshaping the bony orbit. The decision to ablate the sinus is based on the anatomy encountered and leads to 1 of 2 approaches described, type A and type B.

In the type A anatomy, found in approximately 95% of the author's patients, there is a large sinus with pronounced depth and lateral sinus extension accompanied by a large frontonasal duct aperture. For these patients, after the osteotomy and the remodeling of the frontal bone plate are complete, the sinus mucosa is removed and the sinus walls burred out, leaving the frontonasal duct open and functional. The frontal bone plate is then repositioned by impacting it within the sinus cavity to create bone-to-bone contact. Bone chips and bone paste are used to fill in the small gaps and to

contour the brow. The author tries to use either no hardware or at most a 0.2-mm wire when contouring the forehead. The author has not used any titanium mesh in the past 3 years and never miniplates, but these materials can be used without inconvenience if, for instance, if it is necessary to give more stability to the reconstruction and attachment to the frontal bone.

In type B situations (only 5% of the author's cases), the sinus is small and the frontonasal duct less developed. In these patients, the sinus is defunctionalized by burring out the mucosa, ablating the sinus with bone chips, and pasting and then impacting the bone plate on top and sealing it with additional bone paste. Using this algorithmic approach, the author has not had any infections or mucoceles. Finally, what happens after placing the forehead bone flap inside the frontal sinus is that the latter becomes smaller but keeps being permeable. The removal of the mucosa is a technical matter because it is strictly necessary to do it when placing the bone flap inside the frontal sinus.[29–32]

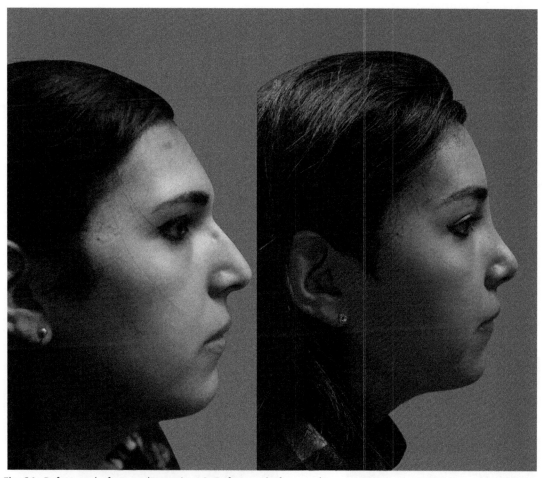

Fig. 24. Before and after results, patient 2. Before and after results.

In addition to changing the approach of the frontal region, the approach to the orbit also has evolved. The classic shaving of the supraorbital rim does not provide a sufficient degree of feminization that many patients desire, so the author performs a more radical reshaping of the orbit using ostectomy of the superolateral orbital rim. The remodeling of the roof and the lateral orbital rim can be included in some cases to soften the appearance, and burring beneath the upper border of the orbital aperture can be used to increase the height of this opening. These maneuvers combine to achieve a greater degree of feminization.

OPERATING LOGISTICS

Many patients come to have full treatment of the face for feminization purposes and facial aging. It is possible to perform a complete FFS and if necessary add a face and neck lift, blepharoplasty, and other aesthetic procedures in the same surgery or to design 2-step surgery separated by a minimum

10 days, so a very long surgery is not performed and in cases of a patient wanting to have all the procedures done in the course of a month. In the first surgical stage, the face and neck lift are done together with the chin and jaw remodeling; this allows having an excellent result due to the great dissection that is generated, plus the lifting is done without causing any edema or inflammation in the face. At the time of the second surgery, the forehead and orbital rim remodeling, hairline correction, brow lift, blepharoplasty, rhinoplasty, and any remaining small procedures are performed (**Figs. 21–24**).

The 1-stage surgery, typically done in a patient who does not require facial rejuvenation procedures, begins with the forehead and orbital rim remodeling, eyebrow lift, and hairline lowering and correction while simultaneously another team begins with the jaw and chin remodeling approach or with the Adam's apple remodeling if necessary. After completion of those procedures, the rhinoplasty, superior lip lift, and the remaining procedures of the lower face can be done.

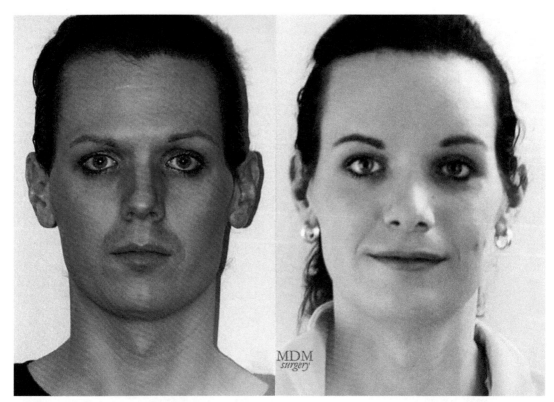

Fig. 25. Before and after results, patient 3. Before and after results.

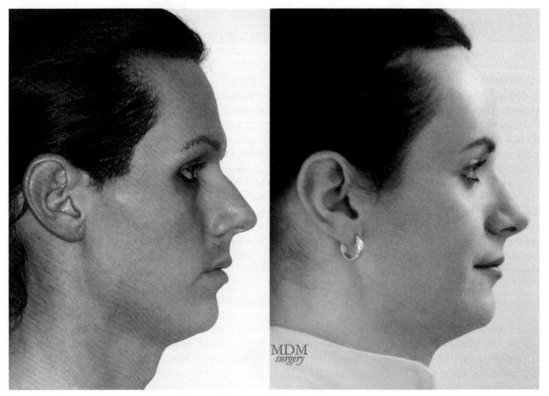

Fig. 26. Before and after results, patient 4. Before and after results.

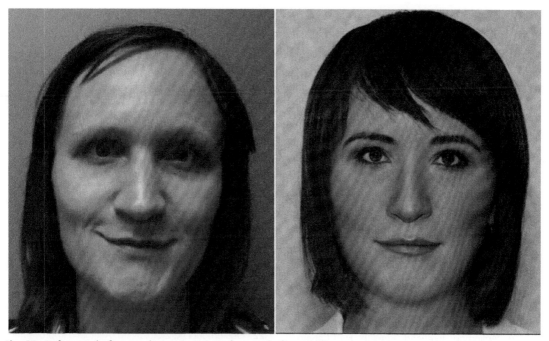

Fig. 27. Before and after results, patient 5. Before and after results.

SUMMARY

Craniofacial surgery has a significant role to play in the treatment of GD and facial features dysphoria. The aim of facial feature remodeling surgery is to project a patient's identity naturally and harmoniously. By simultaneously addressing the bony and soft tissue problems, more dramatic improvements in feminization, as well as rejuvenation, can be achieved. The author has found the modifications in the approach to the fronto-orbital region provide a greater degree of feminization of the periorbital region than was previously able to be

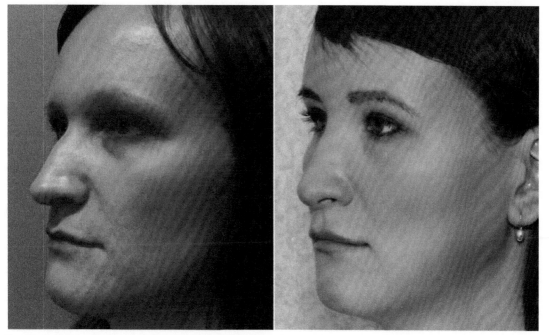

Fig. 28. Before and after results, patient 6. Before and after results.

achieved with traditional techniques and allow comprehensive improvement in a shorter time course than what is typically provided for patients undergoing FFS, without increasing the risk of complications. Without a doubt, the foundation of the feminization and the facial features remodeling is the forehead and orbital rim remodeling together with the remodeling of the frontonasal angle that gives continuity to the rhinoplasty. The orbital rim remodeling surgery to change the expression of the eyes is key to obtain the best result possible (**Figs. 25–28**).

REFERENCES

1. American Psychiatric Association. Diagnostic and statistical manual of mental disorders, fourth edition, text revision. Washington, DC: American Psychiatric Association; 2000.
2. Ricketts RM. Divine proportion in facial esthetics. Clin Plast Surg 1982;9:401–22.
3. Spiegel JH. Facial determinants of female gender and feminizing forehead cranioplasty. Laryngoscope 2011;121:250–61.
4. Ousterhout DK. Feminization of the forehead: contour changing to improve female aesthetics. Plast Reconstr Surg 1987;79:701–13.
5. Farkas LG, Munro IR. Anthropometric facial proportions in medicine. Springfield (IL): Charles C Thomas; 1986.
6. Farkas LG, Kolar JC. Anthropometrics and art in the aesthetics of women's faces. Clin Plast Surg 1987; 14:599.
7. Seghers M, Longacre J, deStefano G. The golden proportion and beauty. Plast Reconstr Surg 1964; 34:241.
8. Vegter F, Hage J. Clinical anthropometry and canons of the face in historical perspective. Plast Reconstr Surg 2000;106:1090.
9. Wolf SA. Application of craniofacial techniques to the everyday practice aesthetic surgery. In: Caronni EP, editor. Craniofacial surgery. Boston: Little, Brown; 1985. p. 507.
10. Ortiz Monasterio F. Aesthetic surgery of the facial skeleton: the forehead. Clin Plast Surg 1991;18:19–27.
11. Marchac D, Durand JL, Renier D. The history of cranioplasty. Ann Chir Plast Esthet 1997;42(1):75–83.
12. Marchac D, Renier D, Arnaud E. Evaluation of the effect of early mobilization of the supraorbital bar on the frontal sinus and frontal growth. Plast Reconstr Surg 1995;95(5):802–11.
13. Molina F. Aesthetic facial osteotomies in latin americans. Clin Plast Surg 2007;34:e31–6.
14. Whitaker LA, Morales L, Farkas LG. Aesthetic surgery of the supraorbital ridge and forehead structures. Plast Reconstr Surg 1986;78(1):23–32.
15. Whitaker LA, Pertschuk M. Facial skeletal contouring for aesthetic purposes. Plast Reconstr Surg 1982; 69(2):245–53.
16. Ortiz Monasterio F. Aesthetic facial osteotomies. In: Terino E, editor. Three dimensional facial sculpting. New York: Informa Healthcare; 2007. p. 219–42.
17. Bartlett SP, Wormon I III, Whitaker L. Evaluation on facial skeletal aesthetics and surgical planning. Clin Plast Surg 1991;18:1–9.
18. Czerwinski M, Hopper RA, Gruss J, et al. Major morbidity and mortality rates in craniofacial surgery: an analysis of 8101 major procedures. Plast Reconstr Surg 2010;126(1):181–6.
19. Whitaker LA. Aesthetic contouring of the facial support system. Clin Plast Surg 1989;16:815.
20. Becking AG, Tuinzing DB, Hage JJ, et al. Facial corrections in male to female transsexuals: a preliminary report on 16 patients. J Oral Maxillofac Surg 1996;54:413–8 [discussion: 419].
21. Becking AG, Tuinzing DB, Hage JJ, et al. Transgender feminization of the facial skeleton. Clin Plast Surg 2007;34:557–64.
22. Ousterhout DK, Zlotolow IM. Aesthetic improvement of the forehead utilizing methylmethacrylate onlay implants. Aesthetic Plast Surg 1990;14:281–5.
23. Mutaz B, Habal MD. Aesthetics of feminizing the male face by craniofacial contouring of the facial bones. Aesthetic Plast Surg 1990;14:143–50.
24. Capitán L, Simon D, Kaye K, et al. Facial feminization surgery: the forehead. Surgical techniques and analysis of results. Plast Reconstr Surg 2014;134:609–19.
25. Spiegel JH. Challenges in care of the transgender patient seeking facial feminization surgery. Facial Plast Surg Clin North Am 2008;16:233–8, viii.
26. Ousterhout DK. Facial feminization surgery: a guide for the transgendered woman. Omaha (Nebraska): Addicus Books; 2009.
27. Ousterhout DK. Facial feminization surgery: the forehead. surgical techniques and analysis of results. Plast Reconstr Surg 2015;5136(4):560e–1e.
28. Whitaker LA, Munro IR, Salyer KE, et al. Combined report of problems and complications in 793 craniofacial operations. Plast Reconstr Surg 1979;64(2): 198–203.
29. Rohrich RJ, Hollier LH. Management of frontal sinus fractures: changing concepts. Clin Plast Surg 1992; 19:219–32.
30. Rohrich RJ, Mickel TJ. Frontal sinus obliteration: in search of the ideal autogenous material. Plast Reconstr Surg 1995;95:580–5.
31. Wolfe SA, Johnson P. Frontal sinus injuries: primary care and management of late complications. Plast Reconstr Surg 1988;82:781–91.
32. Mickel TJ, Rohrich RJ, Robinson JB Jr. Frontal sinus obliteration: a comparison of fat, muscle, bone, and spontaneous osteoneogenesis in the cat model. Plast Reconstr Surg 1995;95:586.

Midfacial Bony Remodeling

Kalle Conneryd Lundgren, MD, PhD*, Maarten J. Koudstaal, MD, DMD, PhD

KEYWORDS

- Craniofacial surgery • Midface surgery • Gender reassignment surgery • Facial feminization surgery

KEY POINTS

- Craniofacial procedures to the midface in conjunction with work to the upper face and skull, and if needed the lower jaw, are a permanent and effective way to achieve feminization of the face in transgender patients.
- This surgery is more complex than other procedures, such as placement of implants and fillers, but should be considered for select patients to achieve a predictable and permanent feminization of the face.
- Cosmetic surgery to the face may be considered a separate surgical entity and is not limited in scope or time by having undergone midface osteotomies.

INTRODUCTION

The face is not as easily dressed or hidden as are other areas of one's physique. In particular, the midface is highly exposed, surrounding the eyes, nose, and mouth, and can hardly be covered by clothing or by a wig, as can be done with the upper part of the skull or a scarf, as can be used for covering up the neck and lower face. Because the face, in most cultures, is essential for interpersonal interactions, an incongruity between one's assigned gender at birth and the appearance of one's face may be severely distressing, and many patients have a strong desire to alleviate this dysphoria by means of physical transition.[1] It is an established fact that patients with gender dysphoria are at increased risk of suffering from minority stress and that this is predictive of psychiatric disorders, such as depression and/or suicidal behavior.[2] Data are growing on the specific importance of the facial structures as they relate to perceived congruence between the experienced gender identity and the bodily appearance.[3–5]

The timing of when a person starts the active gender transition is important for what surgical means may be necessary for altering the facial appearance. In individuals who start transition early in life, counter hormones against testosterone are commonly used and such treatment has a significant impact on the development and further growth of the midfacial structures, as the size and depth of the orbits are nearly final by 6 to 8 years of age and the skull circumference even earlier than that. Other areas with bony bossings, the lower jaw, the nasal bones and cartilage, as well as the overall facial projection and shape, do not complete until after puberty and are highly affected by the presence or absence of testosterone. Consequently, the start of hormonal treatment after the onset of puberty will not prevent the development of facial bony structures with a typical masculine appearance.[6] This is perceived as unwanted in many patients undergoing a

Disclosure Statement: The authors have nothing to disclose.
Declaration of Interests: No conflict of interests for any author.
Department of Craniofacial Diseases, Karolinska University Hospital, Stockholm 171 77, Sweden
* Corresponding author.
E-mail address: kalle.conneryd-lundgren@sll.se

Facial Plast Surg Clin N Am 27 (2019) 221–226
https://doi.org/10.1016/j.fsc.2018.12.004
1064-7406/19/© 2019 Elsevier Inc. All rights reserved.

male-to-female gender transition. Patients transitioning from a female to a male gender are less frequently disturbed by the osteology of the face. Although there are scarce data available on the reasons for the female-to-male group of patients being less distressed by a non–gender-conforming (feminine) osteology of the midface, it may be speculated that there are cultural as well as practical reasons in play. In many modern societies, a certain androgyny among male individuals can be regarded as attractive, compared with the male ideals in commercial campaigns and so forth. Also, the possibility of growing a beard or mustache among female-to-male patients undergoing testosterone supplementation may alleviate any need for other masculinizing maneuvers even in an otherwise rather feminine face.

MIDFACIAL BONY REMODELING FOR FEMINIZING PURPOSES

Facial feminization surgery (FFS) is a collective term to describe the surgical alteration of a masculine facial appearance to a more feminine appearance, most commonly performed for male-to-female transsexual individuals. FFS as a collection of techniques is used to decrease the degree of physical incongruence.[7,8] Several separate surgical techniques have been described and are used under the umbrella of FFS. Among these are placement of implants, fat grafting (lipofilling), injection of artificial substances, such as hyaluronic acid mixtures, as well as surgical work to the bony structures using techniques derived from the field of craniofacial surgery. The broader topic of FFS was recently reviewed by Morrison and colleagues.[9] In this section, we limit discussion to surgery on the midfacial bony structures. Several of the nonbony techniques are rather well established in their use toward performing facial feminizations.[7,8,10] With regard to the midface, skeletal work is less common and fewer data are available in the scientific literature. Mostly implants, fillers, or fat grafting have more often been used for the purpose of augmenting and reshaping the midface. Such approaches are technically less challenging compared with skeletal repositioning, but they may come with the limitations of having to be repeated, as well as a difficult to predict long-term result. The need for repeat surgery when implants or grafting techniques are used are a result of the face's well-known propensity to thin out locally and to "sink" as an effect of gravity when the patient ages. This may result in that the position of an augmented soft tissue area after several years will no longer be appropriate for the patient's

age and that the relative position of the soft tissues and the underlying bone may no longer match. It should also be kept in mind that this is a patient group in whom the purpose of the surgery is not primarily to improve appearance in terms of beauty, but rather to feminize the face. This means that although the same patient may be interested in acquiring a more youthful or beautiful look as they age, this should be regarded by the surgeon as a somewhat separate entity to the feminization aspects of the face. Such reasoning is the basis for providing a long-term plan and result for the patient and to avoid creating what patients have been calling "a trans-appearance." To this end, an improved midfacial osteology will allow the patient to age gracefully, similar to other female individuals. Whether the patient chooses to add cosmetic procedures for aesthetic reasons at one point or another throughout life is then a personal choice.

The overall purpose of FFS surgery as it relates to bony structures is largely to relatively reduce the supraorbital region and orbital rims compared with the overall projection of the patient's midface; this relation has previously been helped by malar implants or lipo filling to the same region.[7,10,11] When surgery to the bone is considered, this relation is first determined based on 3-dimensional (3D) computed tomography (CT) scans and 3D photography, and patients with limited projection at the zygomatic and malar region may be offered bony surgery to augment the projection and angulation of the zygomatic body and inferior orbital rim. In patients who are planned for surgery of the midface, we also perform surgery to reduce the supraorbital ridge and the superior and lateral orbital rims, as described by Capitan and colleagues.[10] This is necessary to create a natural appearance and to avoid distinct transitions between subunits of the face. Many patients also have a typical male configuration with a prominent mentum and/or mandibular lower border and these areas will then be treated for the same reasons. The techniques for treating the lower jaw and mentum area by bony reduction and reshaping has been well described by other investigators.[11] There are similarities in the objectives between the surgical treatment of feminization patients and patients with midfacial retrusion or underdevelopment, such as is often present in patients with craniofacial syndromes. However, the latter group most often has a general underdevelopment or "dish face" appearance, whereas patients undergoing feminization do not. Male-to-female patients rather have particular areas that need increased projection, whereas other nearby areas would benefit from reduced projection. Again, obtaining a good result is all about the relations between bony midfacial structures rather than their absolute positions or measurements. As a result of this, a traditional Le Fort 3 advancement would not be beneficial to FFS patients, as this procedure incorporates the nose, which is not an area that is typically in need of increased projection in FFS patients; in fact, the opposite is most often true. Nor is there normally a need for altering the occlusion in FFS patients, which is in contrast to patients with a congenital underdevelopment of the midface. To selectively augment the zygomas and infraorbital rims, a segmentalized osteotomy approach is indicated. Such an approach was pioneered by Hopper and colleagues[12] for children with Apert syndrome, but for that specific patient group it is used to other ends and different purposes.

Surgery for the FFS patient is performed using a coronal incision that is also the access route for the upper supraorbital rim and the frontal sinus area. These 2 areas are treated first, the anterior frontal sinus wall is released, the bone is thinned by bringing it down and reshaped before placing it back in a more posterior position using titanium fixation. The remaining area of the forehead is then burred down to smooth out the overall contour and to create a more posterior slope from caudal to cranial. The supraorbital rim is burred down to decrease the depth of the upper orbit creating a less deep-set eye position, and this reduction of bone is extended to the upper part of the lateral orbital rim. This has been described by Capitan and colleagues.[10] After having reshaped the upper frontal area of the skull, we would then proceed to the midface part of the procedure. The coronal incision is extended caudally toward each ear as necessary for exposure. An intraoral upper sulcus incision is performed for access to the maxilla and a transconjunctival incision is performed bilaterally and used for access to the inferior orbital margin. Using these incisions, the whole midface is exposed in a subperiosteal plane. The first osteotomies are performed at the zygomatic arch (**Fig. 1**). The position of the osteotomies at the arch should be placed far enough posterior in an area in which the arch is nearly straight and running in a sagittal direction, avoiding steps in the most projected areas. The second osteotomies are done inferior to the frontozygomatic suture at a position just below the area in which the previous burring down was stopped (see **Fig. 1**). To allow for advancement of the infraorbital rim, the previous 2 osteotomies must then be connected using an osteotomy at the medial end of the segment of the zygoma. This osteotomy is commonly placed medial to the infraorbital foramen, as a lateral position may create a step in the inferior orbital rim once repositioned. However, this is somewhat dependent on the patient's specific anatomy and it also may be placed lateral to the nerve, reducing the risk of damaging the nerve itself. The medial osteotomy is performed in a straight vertical angle from the transconjunctival access caudally through the anterior maxillary sinus wall. The connection between the lateral osteotomies at the lateral orbital rim and the medial osteotomy at the inferior orbital rim is performed using a piezoelectric saw, but also can be done using an osteotome or reciprocal saw. To connect the cuts intraorbital, we start on the lateral inner side of the orbit, keeping a few millimeters posterior to the infraorbital margin,

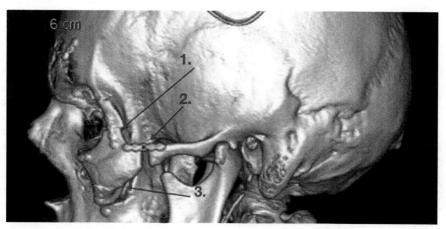

Fig. 1. Computerized tomography, Sagittal view. Osteotomies at the lateral orbital margin (1), zygomatic arch (2), and the posterior wall of the zygoma/maxillary sinus (3).

continue through the orbital floor past the maxillo-zygomatic suture until the medial osteotomy is reached. From intraoral, the anterior wall of the maxilla is then cut further vertically extending the previous medial osteotomy to a point superior to the alveolar ridge and the roots of the teeth. To allow for mobilization, using a saw, an angled cut from medial to lateral passing through the lateral pillar of the maxilla and then through the posterior wall of the maxillary sinus and the posterior part of the zygomatic body is performed to disconnect the whole segment on each side of the face (see **Fig. 1**). To reposition the zygomatic segments, we use titanium plates prebent for the desired position bridging first the osteotomies at the infraorbital rim. Based on the preoperative CT scans, the distance for advancement has been decided, but our experience is that this usually is between 4 and 7 mm. Furthermore, as the maximum projection of the craniofacial skeleton is not in a straight sagittal direction, the bending of the plates also should guide the position of the zygomatic regions to allow for a slight rotation laterally. We usually rotate the segments approximately 3 mm laterally (**Fig. 2**).[13] Once the position is deemed satisfactory, the bones are finally fixed at the zygomatic arch, lateral orbital rim, and medially on the maxilla using titanium micro plates (see **Fig. 1**). We provide all patients with a cooling mask for the first postoperative night and perform a postoperative CT scan. Antibiotics are given as a single dose at the start of surgery. Patients are swollen after surgery, but can usually open their eyes to see well

enough by the first day and most patients can be uneventfully discharged after 1 to 3 days. We do not perform any simultaneous soft tissue surgery, as this is usually not needed and surgery to the nose is done only on esthetic indication. Results are gathered for research using 3D stereophotography surface scanning (**Fig. 3**).

DISCUSSION

Relative projection of distinct areas of the craniofacial skeleton is largely determining the appearance of the facial framework as it relates to a feminine or masculine appearance. It is important to acquire an understanding of the importance of the relative *relations* rather than absolute measurements within the craniofacial skeleton to fully appreciate which regions are in need of treatment, and how, as the objective in FFS surgery is not that of changing an appearance but of feminizing it. Data on relations in the craniofacial skeleton is not readily available in the literature and especially not with regard to male versus female skeletal configurations. This is a shortcoming and means that we currently need to use experience and trial and error using preoperative surgical planning software to determine the best surgical plan. Where the feminization of the upper face is somewhat more straightforward because the objective here is to reduce the supraorbital and frontal sinus protrusion to somewhat of a straight/smooth contour and we do have the rest of the skull as a reference, the midface is more challenging. In the midface, we disconnect large parts of bone and in doing so, we lose reference to the remainder of the bony structures. This means that a clear surgical plan is needed beforehand and prebent plates are often a necessity to not overproject or underproject and to also avoid creating an asymmetry between the facial halves. It should be taken into account that the patient may not be entirely symmetric by nature and a decision then has to be made, together with the patient, on whether symmetry postoperatively is wished for or not. If not, a nonequidistant advancement is needed between the facial sides. The upper and lateral portions of the orbital rims also should be less pronounced than in the typical male individual,[7,10,11] and these are the regions immediately connecting to the midface. In cases in which the patients already have a good projection of the midface, the reduction of the upper facial areas may be able to fully achieve a feminized appearance, as the relative position compared with the zygomatic projections will be posterior enough. The limitation in the amount of bone being possible to remove at the frontal sinus and frontal bone is determined by the thickness of

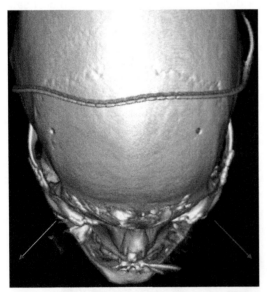

Fig. 2. Computerized tomography, horizontal view. Arrows denote the direction of maximal midface projection.

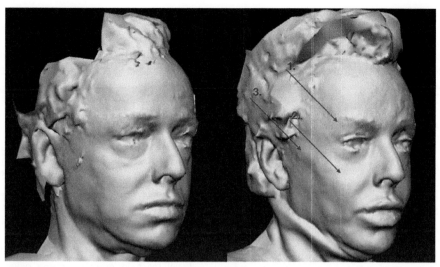

Fig. 3. 3D photography surface scan. Left: preoperative. Right: postoperative. Arrows denote the areas of feminized projection of the midface. (1) Lateral and upper orbital rim, (2) zygomatic body, (3) lateral aspects of the anterior zygomatic arch.

the cortex of the skull and consequently only so much may be reduced. This area then needs to have a smooth connection to the orbital rims, thereby limiting the amount of bone being possible to reduce also at the orbital area, and in a stepwise consequential manner the midface projection is then often needed to be augmented to achieve the desired feminine relations. A significant reduction of the upper facial bones also risks contributing to a dish-face–like look if the midface region is also flat by nature, and this should be taken into account when planning the upper surgery of the face when a midface procedure is not planned. Our decision to perform bony surgery to the midface rather than augmentive work using implants, fillers, or lipo filling is dictated mainly by 2 circumstances. To our knowledge, Sweden is the first country to support FFS for patients with gender dysphoria within public health. This limits us to perform only what can be described as feminizing surgery and not cosmetically driven procedures.[14] This is sometimes not an easily determined distinction, as there can be a blurry line between the desire to look more feminine and to look more beautiful or younger. The other circumstance in our setting is that patients among this group are commonly young and will optimally be treated by surgical means to thereafter live in the desired gender without having to undergo further procedures. They often have a wish to grow old with their feminized face but not have to be seen and treated by public health again for this issue. They do not perceive themselves as ill, and long for a life without frequent health care contacts and appointments. In the long term, the thinning of the soft

tissues and the reduced tone of facial musculature as well as the effects of gravity on the soft tissues often leads to a need for further augmentation of previously augmented areas if the soft tissues rather than the bone have been treated. The approach in which the underlying bone is addressed, rather than masking procedures with the soft tissues, has the clear advantage that aging on the soft tissues follows a natural course. Similarly, if implants on the bone are used, repositioning and exchange of the implants to achieve an appearance adequate for the patient's age may be needed. To this end, we chose to perform bony procedures to the midface for most patients. The repositioned skeleton will undergo the same aging as the remainder of the facial skeleton and hopefully follow-up procedures will be unneeded for feminizing purposes. The feminized bony framework is also a good ground for further cosmetic procedures performed in private care should the patient wish for it.

SUMMARY

We suggest that craniofacial procedures to the midface in conjunction with work to the upper face and skull and if needed the lower jaw is a permanent and effective way to achieve feminization of the face in transgender patients. Although the surgery is more complex than other procedures, such as placement of implants and fillers, it should be considered for select patients. Further improvement of cosmesis may be considered a separate surgical entity and is not limited in scope or time by having undergone midface osteotomies. When carefully planned, bony surgery to the midface using established craniofacial techniques is safe and results in long-term predictive results and a favorable age-appropriate appearance as the patient grows older.

REFERENCES

1. American Psychiatric Association. DSM-5. Available at: http://psychiatry.org/psychiatrists/practice. Accessed October 1, 2018.

2. Rood BA, Puckett JA, Pantalone DW, et al. Predictors of suicidal ideation in a statewide sample of transgender individuals. LGBT Health 2015;2(3):270–5.

3. Dhejne C, Lichtenstein P, Boman M, et al. Long-term follow-up of transsexual persons undergoing sex reassignment surgery: cohort study in Sweden. PLoS One 2011;6(2):e16885.

4. Dhejne C, Van Vlerken R, Heylens G, et al. Mental health and gender dysphoria: a review of the literature. Int Rev Psychiatry 2016;28(1):44–57.

5. Isung J, Möllermark C, Farnebo F, et al. Craniofacial reconstructive surgery improves appearance congruence in male-to-female transsexual patients. Arch Sex Behav 2017;46(6):1573–6.

6. van de Grift TC, Cohen-Kettenis PT, Steensma TD, et al. Body satisfaction and physical appearance in gender dysphoria. Arch Sex Behav 2016;45(3):575–85.

7. Ousterhout DK. Feminization of the forehead: contour changing to improve female aesthetics. Plast Reconstr Surg 1987;79(5):701–13.

8. Altman K. Facial feminization surgery: current state of the art. Int J Oral Maxillofac Surg 2012;41(8):885–94.

9. Morrison SD, Vyas KS, Motakef S, et al. Facial feminization: systematic review of the literature. Plast Reconstr Surg 2016;137(6):1759–70.

10. Capitan L, Simon D, Kaye K, et al. Facial feminization surgery: the forehead. Surgical techniques and analysis of results. Plast Reconstr Surg 2014;134(4):609–19.

11. Becking AG, Tuinzing DB, Hage JJ, et al. Transgender feminization of the facial skeleton. Clin Plast Surg 2007;34(3):557–64.

12. Hopper RA, Kapadia H, Morton T. Normalizing facial ratios in Apert syndrome patients with Le Fort II midface distraction and simultaneous zygomatic repositioning. Plast Reconstr Surg 2013;132(1):129–40.

13. Lundgren TK, Farnebo F. Midface osteotomies for feminization of the facial skeleton. Plast Reconstr Surg Glob Open 2017;5(1):e1210.

14. God vård av vuxna med könsdysfori. Stockholm (Sweden). Socialstyrelsen. Available at: https://www.socialstyrelsen.se/publikationer2015/2015-4-7.

Hair Transplantation Techniques for the Transgender Patient

Anthony Bared, MD*, Jeffrey S. Epstein, MD

KEYWORDS

- Hair transplantation • Transgender • Hair restoration • Hairline patterns

KEY POINTS

- Hairline patterns and facial hair distribution can be gender-identifying traits.
- Women tend to have a lower and more rounded hairline than men as well as more arched brows, whereas men have a prevalence of facial hair.
- Hair transplantation can play a complementary role for the transgender patient undergoing gender transformation.

INTRODUCTION

Hair restoration can play an important role for transgender patients seeking gender transformation procedures.[1–4] The authors' clinic has seen an increase in transgender patients seeking hair restoration. The most common hair restoration procedures performed in the clinic for transgender patients are hairline lowering procedures; facial hair restoration procedures, including eyebrow and beard transplantation; and, less frequently, body hair transplantation. Hair restoration can be an important component for male-to-female (MTF) transgender patients as part of the gender transformation because the rounding of a hairline, for instance, can help provide for a more feminine appearance as does creating an arched shape to the eyebrows. For female-to-male (FTM) patients, beard and chest hair transplantation helps create a more masculine facial and body appearance. This article presents the authors' experience in hair restoration for transgender patients. The best candidates for hair restoration as it relates to transgender patients, the techniques that provide for the most natural results, and the postoperative course from hair transplantation are reviewed.

PREOPERATIVE PLANNING
Consultation

The consultation for hair restoration serves to attain a medical and hair loss history, to ascertain a patient's goals for the procedure, to provide for a proper examination of the scalp donor hair and recipient area, and to establish mutual goals for the procedure. A hair loss–specific questionnaire is completed by the patient prior to the consultation and this is reviewed with the patient at the time of consultation. Hair loss history needs to be obtained if there is androgenic hair loss evident in the patient as well as a family history of hair loss. In the MTF patient taking hormonal therapy or having undergone gender reassignment, there is no further risk of potential future male pattern hair loss. Examination of the scalp, paying close attention to the quality of the donor hair, needs to be performed. The donor hair needs to be examined for its quality and density so as to estimate the number of grafts that may be obtained in a procedure as well as over the course of the patient's lifetime. When reviewing the patient's goals for the procedure, whether hairline lowering or facial hair restoration, it is often helpful that the patient brings model photos of their ideal outcome to

Disclosure Statement: The authors have nothing to disclose.
Private Practice, Foundation for Hair Restoration, 6280 Sunset Drive, Suite 504, Miami, FL, USA
* Corresponding author.
E-mail address: abared@dranthonybared.com

Facial Plast Surg Clin N Am 27 (2019) 227–232
https://doi.org/10.1016/j.fsc.2018.12.005

review at the time of the consultation. The authors do not perform computerized imaging for hair restoration, finding that this gives unrealistic expectations from surgery, but instead marks out photos of patients, drawing in for them the potential position of their hairline or beard shape. As in any area of aesthetic surgery, proper expectations need to be established and understood, whether the degree of hairline lowering possible through a single procedure or the amount of density attainable in either hairline lowering or facial hair restoration. Risks of the procedure are reviewed with the patient. Lastly, patients need to be in generally good medical health to undergo a procedure.

Hairline Design

Although hairline designs vary tremendously, the important goal is that of achieving a natural-appearing female hairline. When designing a hairline for the transgender patient, multiple factors need to be considered. The position of the existing hairline, the presence of androgenic alopecia, family history of hair loss, use of hormonal therapy such as finasteride or estrogens, and the density and quality of the donor hair are all factors to keep in mind. In general, feminizing a hairline entails the lowering of the hairline and the blunting of the temporal region. A soft, heart-shaped hairline design with rounded recession in the frontal-temporal region (**Fig. 1**) is often used to feminize the hairline and achieve a natural appearance to the hairline. To aid in the creation of a natural hairline appearance, often a subtle widow's peak is created slightly off-center. Rounding of the hairline is then performed posteriorly and laterally along the frontal-temporal region, connecting to the temporal points. This design helps soften the hairline,

blunt the temporal area, and feminize the hairline. On the day of the procedure, the patient is met in the preoperative suite where her hairline is marked out using a washable surgical marking pen. The hairline is inspected for symmetry. The patient is then shown the hairline design in front of a mirror. Once the hairline design is agreed on, the markings are reinforced with a more permanent-inked marker so as not to wash off during the procedure. Preoperative photos are taken before and after the markings.

Beard Design

Goals in beard design are often established by the patient. Many patients typically present with a specific understanding of how they want their facial hair to appear. The design and density of the beard may be limited by the quality of the donor hair. Transplantation of full beards requires large amount of grafts, and patients are always made aware of the possibility of undergoing secondary procedures after approximately 1 year if further density is desired. It is the authors' experience that the scalp hair transplants to the face have a high regrowth percentage and, if properly performed, patients can achieve a natural outcome. Depending on the exact design and density, graft counts can range from 250 to 300 grafts to each sideburn, 400 to 800 grafts to the mustache and goatee, and 300 to 500 grafts per cheek. Using the patient's guidelines, the areas to be transplanted are marked out using a surgical marking pen with the patient in a seated position. The markings are checked for symmetry between the 2 sides. Measurements are used to help ensure symmetry. The patient is shown the markings in a mirror, because the 2-D perspective provided by a mirror, which is what the patient sees, is different than what the surgeon sees in direct 3-D. If needed, alterations are made according to patient desires (**Fig. 2**).

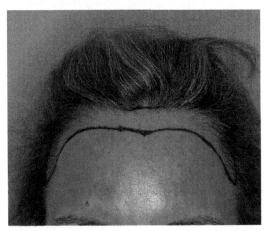

Fig. 1. Female hairline design generally follows a heart-shaped design with slight rounding in the frontal-temporal region.

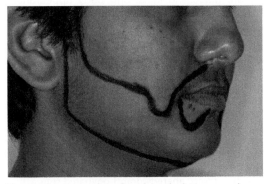

Fig. 2. An example of a beard design as drawn preoperatively.

Eyebrow Design

When approaching eyebrow restoration for the transgender patient, it is important to appreciate the shape of the more masculine eyebrow versus that of a more feminine eyebrow appearance. The masculine eyebrow shape is generally less arched but comes to a lateral widening at the peak of the brow, whereas the feminine eyebrow shape is more rounded and arched (**Fig. 3**). The goal in eyebrow restoration for the transgender patient wishing to create a more feminine appearance is to create a more arched-shaped appearance to the eyebrows, whereas in all patients the goals are to provide the desired shape, density, natural direction, and angle of growth of eyebrow hair. Patients are encouraged to bring in photos of their ideal or model eyebrows. On the day of the procedure, the patient is first seen in the preoperative suite where photos are taken. Preoperative photography is important in eyebrow transplantation because it truly helps provide another means of visualizing the planned eyebrow shape prior to the procedure. Photos are taken of the patient both with eyes open and eyes closed. It is often found that eyebrow elevation is asymmetric, because there tends to be an asymmetric elevation of the eyebrows by the facial musculature and sometimes that associated with asymmetry of the eyelids. These asymmetries are noted and made known to the patient. Most female patients are accustomed to drawing in the eyebrows with an eyeliner pen so they are encouraged to do so at this time in front of a mirror. Once preliminary drawings are made by the patient, the surgeon fine-tunes the shape. Measurements are taken along the length and in various places along the width of the eyebrows to ensure as much symmetry as possible. The midline is marked and measurements off the midline also are taken. The final shape is then shown to the patient, and photos of this shape are taken in a fashion similar to the premarking photos.

SURGICAL PROCEDURE
Donor Hair Harvest

In a majority of all hair transplants the authors perform, the donor hairs are harvested by the follicular unit extraction (FUE) technique, which avoids altogether a linear donor site incision and thus patients typically are able to cut the hair as short as desired. The authors still occasionally use, however, particularly in women, including MTF transgender hair transplants, the strip method for harvesting the donor hairs. The strip method avoids the need for significant shaving of the back and sometimes sides of the head that is typically needed for large FUE procedures. The authors also use, however, a no-shave FUE technique, where the donor hair is extracted via the FUE method while the surrounding hairs in the donor area are maintained long and not needed to be entirely trimmed. This is a more tedious procedure but allows for FUE extraction, avoiding a linear scar, and for patients to maintain their hair long.

Hairline

The position and shape of the hairline are, at first, drawn for the patient using a removable ink marking pen. The patient is shown the hairline design in front of a mirror. Once the position and shape of the hairline are determined, photos are taken of the design and the markings are reinforced with a permanent ink marker so as not to be lost during the procedure. Most patients are then given oral anxiolytic medication.

The goal of hairline lowering is to create the most natural-appearing results by replicating the direction and angle of the existing hairline. The smallest possible incisions are made, allowing for the placement of the hair grafts. The 1-hair, 2-hair, and 3-hair grafts are tested to ensure size compatibility with the recipient sites. Acute angulation of the grafts is important, particularly in the first few rows of the hairline. Depending on the characteristics of the hair—thickness and curl—typically the first 2 to 3 rows are composed of single-hair grafts placed in an irregular pattern, followed by the placement of 2-hair to 3-hair grafts. The central portion of the hairline is the area that tends to be most dense, so it is important that the central aspect is adequately filled to allow for creation of the most density in this region. As

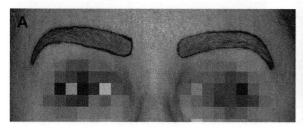
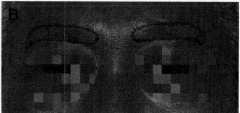

Fig. 3. (*A*) Female eyebrow design. (*B*) Male eyebrow design with a lateral widening and a nonarched design.

discussed previously, the direction of hair growth follows the existing hairline but, most commonly, hairs are placed with an acute forward direction on the central region and then tapered down/inferiorly along the temples (**Fig. 4**). The grafts are then placed in the incisions with implanter devices that minimize trauma to the grafts and can expedite the planting process.

Patients are instructed to expect swelling along the forehead and eyes for 1 day to 2 days after the procedure. They are seen in the office on postoperative day 1 for a hair wash and are instructed how to wash the hair and care for the grafts. Light washings are performed without allowing the shower water to directly hit the grafts for the first 6 days after surgery, followed by normal showers after that point. The crusts are to be gently removed after 6 days.

Beard

Currently in the authors' practice, nearly all patients seeking facial hair restoration elect to have the grafts obtained via the FUE technique. In these cases, the donor area is shaved (unless a no-shave approach is used) and patients are placed in a supine position. The smallest possible drill size, avoiding graft transection, is used for the extractions. The donor area consists of the occiput only in smaller cases and extends into the parietal scalp for larger cases. Once the extractions have been completed from the occipital area, the patient is turned to lie in the supine position.

Local anesthesia is then applied to the face, starting in each sideburn and cheek area. The perioral region is not anesthetized at this point; rather, the area around the mouth is typically worked on after the patient has eaten lunch. The recipient sites in the sideburn and cheek area are made first. The smallest possible recipient sites are made using 0.5-mm, 0.6-mm, and sometimes 0.7-mm slits. In the periphery of the sideburns, 1-hair grafts are used whereas 2-hair grafts can be placed in the central aspect of the sideburn to allow for more density. It is imperative to make the incisions at an ultra-acute angle to the skin. The direction of growth is generally downward but more centrally, closer to the mouth/goatee region, can be somewhat anterior. In the cheek area, mostly 1-hair and 2-hair grafts are used; however, in the occasional patient with fine donor hair, some 3-hair grafts can be used to allow for the achievement of greater density. As soon as recipient site formation is done, the grafts can be placed 1 at a time, according to the vision of the surgeon.

After the patient is given lunch, the area around the mouth is anesthetized. Infraorbital and mental nerve blocks are used to provide initial anesthesia. The goatee and mustache areas' anesthesia are then reinforced with field subdermal local anesthesia complemented by epinephrine 1:50,000 to minimize bleeding. Incisions in the goatee and mustache areas are then made. On the mustache, hairs grow slightly laterally and transition downward along the goatee. Again, it is important to make these at an angle as acute as possible to the skin. The grafts in the mustache region have the tendency to grow perpendicular; thus, patients need to be made aware of the difficulty in creating density along the entire mustache, particularly centrally within the cupid's bow. The creation of density in this area is difficult owing to the topography created by the upper lip's cupid's bow area. The transition from the mustache to the goatee is an important area for the creation of density, which is usually created by the maximal dense packing of 2-hair grafts.

Graft placement continues, and, toward the conclusion of the case, the patient is given a mirror before all grafts are placed. Given that the immediate results closely replicate the final results, it is helpful for the patient to view the beard to assess the design and density of the grafts. This allows for feedback, fine-tuning, and alteration before the conclusion of the case (**Fig. 5**).

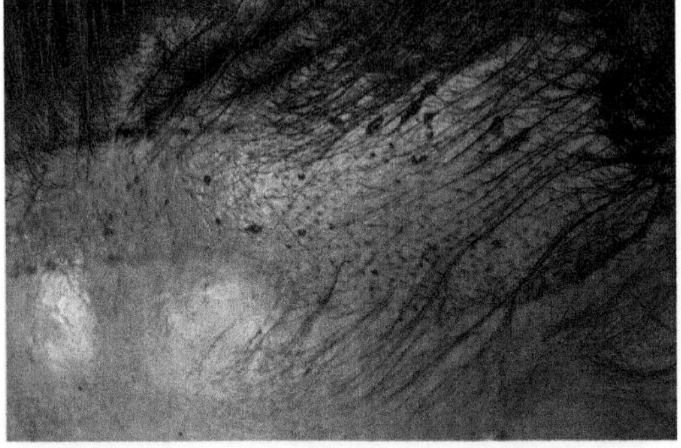

Fig. 4. Intraoperative photo of the direction and angulation of the female hairline graft placement.

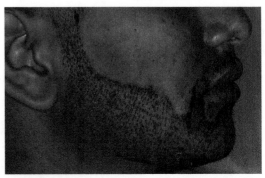

Fig. 5. Immediate, postoperative photo of the patient in **Fig. 2**, showing beard hair graft placement.

Patients are to keep the face dry for the first 5 days after the procedure. This allows the grafts to set properly, helping assure the maintenance of proper angulation. Topical antibiotic ointment is applied to the donor area whether a strip or FUE technique was used. Patients then wet the face after 5 days with soap and water, starting to remove the dried blood and crusts. Shaving is permitted after 10 days.

Eyebrow

The donor area is anesthetized with local anesthesia composed of lidocaine 2%/epinephrine 1:100,000. These grafts can be obtained by the strip or FUE technique. Given the small number of grafts needed for eyebrow transplantation, the no-shave FUE technique can easily be used for those patients electing to not have the strip method while allowing the surrounding hair to be maintained long.

Once the donor hairs have been harvested, the patient is placed in a seated, reclined position for incision site formation. The eyebrow area is anesthetized with local anesthesia containing epinephrine for hemostasis. The recipient sites are made using the smallest blade size for the graft—typically 0.5 mm or 0.6 mm. Initial recipient sites are made along the periphery along the premarked borders of the eyebrows. It is important to start with these peripheral marking incisions because the preoperative markings can soon be lost with subsequent bleeding and wiping. Incisions are made at an angle as acute as possible to the skin (**Fig. 6**). Within the medial-most aspect of the eyebrow inferiorly, the hairs usually grow in a superior and slightly lateral direction. While moving more superior within the head of the eyebrow, the direction changes to a more lateral and then inferior direction. Moving more laterally into the body (midportion), the hairs grow in an inferior-lateral direction along the superior border and in a superior-lateral direction along the inferior border. Within this body, which constitutes the majority of the eyebrow, this crossed-hatch pattern achieves the greatest amount of density. Then, the lateral-most approximately one-quarter of the eyebrow, called the tail, has typically horizontally oriented recipient sites.

Once all incision sites are made, the grafts are inserted. A typical procedure can range from 150 grafts to as many as 400 grafts per eyebrow. The grafts are placed so that the direction of the hair growth, that is, the curl of the hair, is placed to complement the goal of having the hairs grow in an angle as acute as possible with the skin. In most cases, as many 2-hair grafts as possible are placed within the eyebrows, primarily the central portion but also in parts of the head. Two-hair grafts are not used if the hairs within a graft are divergent in their growth. The utilization of as many 2-hair grafts as possible creates the most amount of density within the eyebrows. Mostly 1-hairs grafts are used along the borders, periphery, and tail region. After all the grafts are placed, the patient is asked to sit up and the eyebrows are inspected. Additional grafts are placed if small adjustments are deemed appropriate. The patient is then shown the eyebrows in a mirror for feedback (**Fig. 7**).

Patients are instructed to maintain the eyebrow area dry for 5 days. The scalp hair may be washed the first postoperative day. Antibiotic ointment is applied to the donor area twice daily for 1 week. Patients are allowed to use makeup in the eyebrow area after all the crusts have fallen out, at typically 5 days to 7 days.

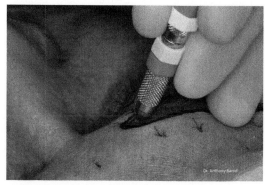

Fig. 6. Incisions are made in an acute angle to the skin with 0.5-mm to 0.6-mm blades.

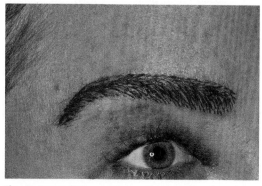

Fig. 7. Immediate, postoperative results of eyebrow transplantation.

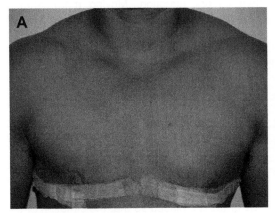
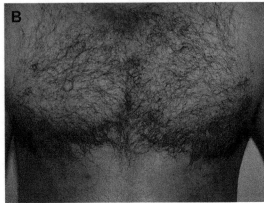

Fig. 8. Before and after 2000 grafts to chest—FTM patient—to create a more masculine appearance and conceal mastectomy scars.

Chest and Other Pubic Region

There are a variety of indications for performing these body hair procedures. Chest hair procedures can serve both to create a more masculine appearance and to help conceal mastectomy scars in MTF patients. Pubic hair transplants are indicated primarily in patients who have undergone gender reassignment, where the normal escutcheon can similarly help conceal any scarring (**Fig. 8**).

For the chest, procedures of 1800 grafts to as many as 3000 grafts are indicated, due to the large area that needs to be covered. These potential areas, depending on patient goals, can include the upper and central chest, ranging laterally and inferiorly (particularly to conceal mastectomy scars) and even continuing caudally in a vertical direction into the abdomen and even upper pubic region. The keys to achieving a natural result, besides careful acute angulation of the recipient sites, is to have a crossed-hatch pattern of hair growth toward the midline, that is, the sternum.

A crossed-hatch pattern centrally—to achieve the greatest appearance of density—is also indicated when performing pubic hair transplants. Typical procedures range from 400 grafts to 900 grafts, depending on a patient's goals in terms of density and area covered.

SUMMARY

Hairline patterns and facial hair distribution can be gender-identifying traits. Women tend to have a lower and more rounded hairline than men as well as having more arched brows, whereas men have a prevalence of facial hair. Hair transplantation can play a complementary role for transgender patients undergoing gender transformation. In the authors' clinic, the most common hair transplantations seen in transgender patients are hairline lowering, beard transplantation, and eyebrow transplantation. Although challenging from artistic and technical perspectives, these procedures have a high satisfaction rate for patients.

REFERENCES

1. Rogers N. Imposters of androgenic alopecia. Facial Plast Surg Clin North Am 2013;21:325–34.
2. Rassman WR, Pak JP, Kim J, et al. Phenotype of normal hairline maturation. Facial Plast Surg Clin North Am 2013;21:317–24.
3. Nausbaum BP, Fuentefria S. Naturally occurring female hairline patterns. Dermatol Surg 2009;35: 907–13.
4. Rassman WR, Berstein RM, McClellan R, et al. Follicular unit extraction: minimally invasive surgery for hair transplantation. Dermatol Surg 2002;28: 720–8.

Lower Jaw Recontouring in Facial Gender-Affirming Surgery

Shane D. Morrison, MD, MS[a],*, Thomas Satterwhite, MD[b,1]

KEYWORDS

- Transgender • Mandible contouring • Lower jaw augmentation • Jaw implants • Osteotomies

KEY POINTS

- Facial gender-affirming surgery can lead to significant improvement in quality-of-life for gender-dysphoric patients.
- Lower jaw feminization consists of bony contouring of mandibular angle and body along with sliding genioplasty.
- Lower jaw masculinization consists of placement of alloplastic implants, fat or bone grafts along the mandibular angle and body, and placement of alloplastic implants or fat along the chin or sliding genioplasty.
- Complications are rare, but can be significant in the setting of nerve injuries, surgical site infections, or implant infections.
- Further research is needed on facial gender-affirming surgery, especially related to patient-reported outcomes.

INTRODUCTION

Gender dysphoria develops from the incongruity between one's assigned sex at birth and one's inherent gender identity.[1] Treatment for gender dysphoria comes in many different forms, from mental health to exogenous hormones to surgical intervention, and all fall under the realm of gender-affirming care.[2] With proper treatment, gender-dysphoric patients endorse decreased psychosocial sequelae and improved quality of life.[3–13] Gender dysphoria can affect a wide range of persons, including transgender, gender nonconforming, gender queer, pangender, and agender populations, among others.[14,15] Globally, the number of transgender people exceeds 25 million and trends in gender-affirming surgery are rising within the United States.[16,17]

Because of significant stigma and discrimination, many of those suffering from gender dysphoria are not able to obtain the care they need, and in some cases this may be related to medical provider knowledge and comfort.[17] Further training on gender-affirming care is needed for physicians, and we are making progress.[18–24] The World Professional Association for Transgender Health (WPATH) develops Standards of Care as guidelines for gender-affirming treatment.[1] Continued enhancement in education and awareness will allow for improved multidisciplinary teams to address gender affirmation.[25]

Disclosure: Authors have no disclosures to declare.
[a] Division of Plastic Surgery, Department of Surgery, University of Washington School of Medicine, 325 9th Avenue Mailstop #359796, Seattle, WA 98104, USA; [b] Brownstein and Crane Surgical Services, San Francisco, CA, USA
[1] Present address: 575 Sr. Francis Drake Boulevard, Suite 1, Greenbrae, CA 94904.
* Corresponding author.
E-mail address: shanedm@uw.edu

Facial Plast Surg Clin N Am 27 (2019) 233–242
https://doi.org/10.1016/j.fsc.2019.01.001

Gender-affirming surgery options for transgender men (female-to-male) include facial, chest, body, and genital masculinization.[6,8,26] Options for transgender women (male-to-female) include facial, vocal, chest, body, and genital feminization.[2,10,11,27] In transmen, the most common surgical procedures are related to chest and body masculinization, whereas transwomen more commonly seek facial, body, and chest feminization.[11,27,28] Pioneering work by Douglas Ousterhout, MD, determined aspects of the craniofacial skeleton that depicted more masculine or feminine features, and this has led to the development of facial gender-affirming surgery.[29-31]

The generally accepted differences between the masculine and feminine faces are numerous. Overall, a feminine face is rounded and soft-appearing with a heart or inverted triangle shape (apex of the triangle at chin and base at malar region), whereas a masculine face is angulated and square with a pronounced jaw and chin. An M-shaped hairline with temporal recession constitutes a more masculine shape. An acute nasofrontal angle, presence of a supraorbital ridge (forehead bossing), and straight eyebrows that sit along the superior orbital rim constitute a

masculine appearance, whereas a gentle curving convex forehead with laterally peaked eyebrows sitting above the superior orbital rim are more feminine. A wide and straight nose with a minimal supratip break is more masculine compared with a thin-based and concave nose. Thin and elongated upper lips further accentuate masculine features. In the lower third of the face, a long, square chin with a prominent mandible with bulky masseter musculature and a sharp mandibular angle are more masculine. Last, a prominent thyroid cartilage with a 90° angle, as opposed to a 120° angle, signals masculinity.[6,11,27,29,31-44] Cultural background may alter one's perception of masculinity and femininity[45] (**Fig. 1**).

Various studies have tried to quantify aspects of the face that more substantially determine masculinity or femininity, yet evaluation of the complete harmonious face has proven the most effective in expressing gender.[11,44] In this article, we discuss contouring of the lower jaw for feminization or masculinization in gender-affirming surgery. Preoperative evaluation and planning, operative techniques, and postoperative care and outcomes are discussed. Some of the techniques discussed have not been published widely and used in only

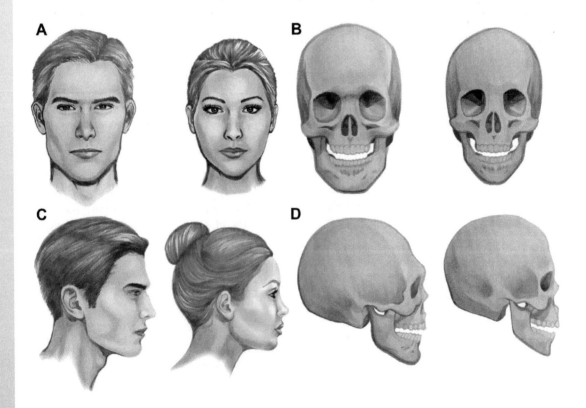

Fig. 1. Difference in male and female faces. (*A*) Frontal soft tissue view. (*B*) Frontal skeletal view. (*C*) Lateral soft tissue view. (*D*) Lateral skeletal view. (*Courtesy of* Thomas Satterwhite, MD.)

a few patients (facial masculinization), whereas others are better known (facial feminization).

PREOPERATIVE ASSESSMENT

Before surgery, all patients have a preoperative evaluation with the surgical team. There are no guidelines set forth by the WPATH for patients who wish to have facial gender-affirming surgery.[1] For our patients, we generally prefer them to have met with a mental health provider who can evaluate their gender dysphoria and treat any concomitant mental health issues. Likewise, prior hormone therapy is preferred, but not a criterion for consultation or surgery. When possible, we prefer our patients to take hormones for a year before surgery, as we feel this appropriately allows remodeling and texturizing of the soft tissues to approximate what their facial skin will be like as their true gender. An evaluation by a primary care provider for underlying medical conditions (eg, diabetes, congestive heart failure, chronic obstructive pulmonary disease, previous myocardial infarction) that could adversely affect surgical outcomes is needed.

Evaluation by dentistry and orthodontics is important before undertaking lower jaw recontouring. Treatment of underlying caries or gingival disease is needed to prevent potential infection of the surgical sites or the rare, but devastating, risk of osteomyelitis.[4] Evaluation of occlusion and interdental relationships are necessary. Appropriate jaw alignment along with the quality of the teeth can have dramatic effects on perceptions of beauty and gender, so these must be evaluated by the surgeon if the patient is has not seen dentistry or orthodontics before facial gender-affirming surgery consultation.[32,40,46,47] Edentulous mandibles also can place the patient at considerable risk for iatrogenic fractures or nonunions due to the quality of the bone. Presence of impacted third molars or unerupted third molars could affect osteotomy sites, so these also must be evaluated.

During the initial consultation, the surgeon should evaluate the entire face to determine which qualities are feminine and masculine, taking into account patient perceptions of their masculine and feminine aspects. Dividing the face into vertical thirds is a common approach used to investigate the various areas of the face, but the ultimate goal should be a harmonious face that portrays the patient's desired gender. During specific evaluation of the lower third of the face, it is important to evaluate the prominence, splay, and angularity of the mandible and associated masseter muscle bulk, along with the position,

projection, and angularity of the chin. Feminine features include a narrow, short, and pointed chin with narrow and more rounded mandibular angles. Soft tissue draping and laxity with associated rhytids should be noted, especially if platysmal banding or marionette lines are present, as changes to the bony architecture could accentuate or modify these.

Plain radiographs, cephalograms, or computed tomography imaging is optional, but can help with assessment of potential concomitant osteotomies of the midface or supraorbital bossing reduction. It is common that patients seeking facial gender-affirming surgery have multiple procedures performed during a single operation, so these preoperative images allow for planning.[31,42] Photographs should be taken according to accepted standards of the face (1 m from the patient with 105-mm lens) and appropriate modifications for the brow or nose.

Procedures to be performed and their associated risks should be disclosed at consultation. Specifically, risks of infection, injury to tooth roots, and injury to mental or inferior alveolar nerves should be discussed in relation to lower jaw recontouring. Postoperative oral hygiene, diet, and dressings are reviewed at this consultation. Finally, shared decision-making between the patient and the surgeon should assist with the development of final surgical plans.

If deemed an appropriate candidate for surgery, patients must stop taking estrogen and progesterone-based hormones 2 weeks before surgery to minimize the risk of a deep vein thrombosis or pulmonary embolism. Patients may continue to take androgen blockers. Aspirin, antiplatelet agents, and anti-inflammatory agents should be stopped 1 week before surgery. Herbal medications should be reviewed with the patient because many can increase bleeding risk.

SURGICAL APPROACH
Lower Jaw Feminization

Most studies for facial feminization focus on modification of the upper and middle thirds of the face.[29,33,35,36,39–41,45,47–51] Modification of the lower jaw for feminization consists of osteotomies or burring of the mandibular angle to soften the angularity and sliding genioplasty to narrow and decrease the height of the chin.[11,34,52]

As modification of the lower jaw is generally coupled with other procedures for facial feminization, patients are intubated orally, and the endotracheal tube is wired to the maxillary molars with a 26-gauge wire. Care is taken to ensure ventilation is maintained with flexion and extension of the neck before starting the case. The teeth are cleaned with chlorhexidine, and a throat pack is placed to minimize swallowing of blood or other fluids. Cefazolin is given 30 to 60 minutes before the procedure. Antibiotics are re-dosed appropriately during the case. Appropriate warming, deep vein thrombosis prophylaxis with sequential compression devices, and glucose control are applied (**Fig. 2**).

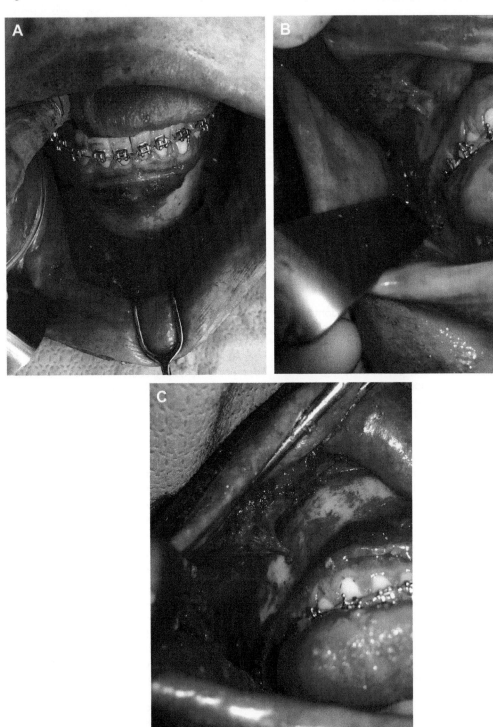

Fig. 2. Mandibular feminization. (*A*) Intraoperative exposure of the entire mandible with exposure and protection of the mental nerves. (*B*) Mandibular angle being smoothed with rasp after burring. (*C*) Mandibular angle and body after contouring.

Mandibular angle recontouring

Local anesthetic is given along the course of the incision from angle to angle. An incision with Bovie electrocautery is made along the area demarcated from the local anesthetic. The incision is placed wide on the gingival mucosa to ensure an adequate cuff of mucosa remains for closure. A cuff of mentalis muscle is left over the symphysis for resuspension during closure to reduce the risk of witch's chin deformity. When combined with genioplasty, the entire soft tissue is stripped off the anterior portion of the mandible in a subperiosteal plane, with care taken to protect the mental nerves. Exposure of the entire lower border of the angle, body, and ramus is paramount to prevent injury to the pterygo-masseteric musculature when performing contouring of the mandible. Langenbecks are placed to ensure wide exposure of the mandibular angle. Oftentimes the angle can be contoured sufficiently with the use of a round or pineapple burr at high speed. Burring of the entire mandible may need to be performed for maximal contouring. Particular attention should be paid to the body of the mandible, which can be quite protrusive in some patients. With removal of the cortical bone and exposure of the cancellous bone, it is important to avoid exposure of the molar roots and inferior alveolar nerve. The burr is used to taper the contoured angle into the mandibular body. When the angle is sufficiently prominent, osteotomies are warranted. Reciprocating, oscillating, or piezoelectric saws are used to perform the initial cuts at the cortical bone. A right angle or curved osteotome completes the osteotomy. Because of the attachment of the medial pterygoid, the fragment can translocate medially and needs to be digitally reduced so the muscle can be divided and the bone extracted. If an osteotomy is done, then the lower border should still be burred to contour the angle. If preoperative analysis suggests excessive masseter bulk, then neurotoxin injection or masseteric resection can be offered. However, masseter atrophy also may occur in the setting of stripping of the mandible, so reduction of the muscle is not a requirement.[32] Hemostasis is achieved, especially if injury occurred to the pterygo-masseteric musculature during angle reduction. Thrombin, gel foam, or other hemostatic agents can be used to assist. If performed in isolation, then the incision can be closed with Chromic or Vicryl suture in a watertight fashion to prevent pooling of saliva. If a concomitant genioplasty is to be performed, the attention is shifted to this procedure.

Sliding genioplasty

When performed with the mandible angle reduction, the incision described previously can be used. If performed in isolation, a labial sulcus incision with a wide cuff of mucosa and cuff of mentalis is performed. Dissection of the anterior mandible is performed in a subperiosteal plane with care taken to avoid the mental nerves. The lower border is stripped of its soft tissue attachments. Once exposed, a line 5 mm below the mental nerves bilaterally is marked. Based on preoperative evaluation, width, height, projection, and asymmetries are addressed. A reciprocating saw is used to make the initial cut for the osteotomy and it is completed with an osteotome. If vertical height is to be reduced, the predetermined amount of bone to be resected is marked, and the osteotomy should be performed initially on the lower line, then the superior line. An oscillating saw is then used to remove a predetermined segment of bone in the midline to allow for narrowing of the chin. The bony segments are collapsed medially and fixed temporarily with wires if needed. The segments are set back a predetermined amount for vertical reduction and fixated with plates and screws. The junction between the posterior genioplasty segments and the mandible should be inspected and palpated to ensure there are no step-offs. To ensure a smooth transition, this area should be burred if needed. Once stable, the incisions are irrigated and closed in layers with Vicryl to resuspend the mentalis, then either Vicryl or Chromic to close the mucosa in a horizontal mattress fashion (**Fig. 3**).

Lower Jaw Masculinization

Only 2 studies have reported on facial masculinization, and only a single study was used for a transman.[31,37] In general, many of the procedures can be thought of as pursuing the opposite of feminization, with augmentation of the bony architecture with implants or the use of malleable material.[53] As these procedures are performed infrequently, some of the steps for these procedures are gleaned from the non-transgender patient-based literature.[31,54,55]

Mandibular angle recontouring

Local anesthetic is given along the course of the incision from angle to angle. An incision is made along the area demarcated from the local anesthetic. The incision is placed wide on the gingival mucosa to ensure a large cuff of mucosa remains for closure. A cuff of mentalis muscle is left over the symphysis for resuspension during closure to reduce the risk of witch's chin deformity. When combined with genioplasty, the entire soft tissue is stripped off the anterior portion of the mandible in a subperiosteal plane, with care taken to protect the mental nerves. Exposure of the entire lower border of the angle, body, and ramus is paramount

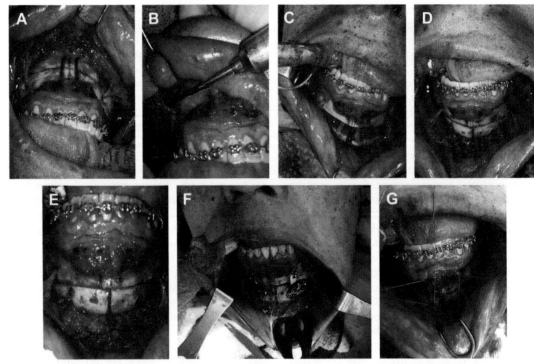

Fig. 3. Sliding genioplasty for feminization. (*A*) Markings for sliding genioplasty illustrating transverse line for horizontal osteotomy and vertical lines for width reduction. (*B*) Horizontal osteotomy being initiated with reciprocating saw. (*C*) Completion of horizontal osteotomy with down-fracturing. (*D*) Inset of chin after horizontal and vertical translation and reduction. (*E*) Placement of screw fixation. (*F*) Alternate fixation of sliding genioplasty with plates. (*G*) Closure of mentalis before mucosal closure.

to prevent injury to the pterygo-masseteric musculature when placing implants, yet when an interposition bone graft is to be placed, then care must be taken to leave the masseter attachments for vascular supply to the bone.

Langenbecks are placed to ensure wide exposure of the mandibular angle when implants are placed. Implants are designed to produce a squarer jaw and are tapered appropriately along the mandibular body to the genioplasty segment (if one is being performed). Care should be taken in their insertion to minimize contamination from intraoral bacteria. The implants are fixed with monocortical screws to the mandible and a watertight closure is needed to prevent saliva pooling on the implants. Most surgeons tend to favor Medpor implants for the angle.

Iliac crest or calvarial bone graft can be harvested through standard means to augment the mandibular angle. Dr Ousterhout pioneered this procedure.[31] He noted that placement of a bone graft between the masseter and lateral cortex of the mandible results in resorption of the bone, so the graft is placed between the medial two-thirds and lateral one-third of the mandible. The approach and technique for a sagittal split

osteotomy is used with 2 important considerations: (1) the mandible remains intact with an intact arch and continuity of condyle with dental segment, and (2) the masseter muscle is not stripped from its insertion. The split is made almost completely with a reciprocating saw and finished with an osteotome, leaving the pterygomandibular ligament intact on the lower border of the mandible. Up to 6 mm of bone graft have been placed. The interposition graft is stabilized between the portions of the mandible without fixation.

A less invasive approach involves fat transfer along the mandible to increase width and projection of the lower face; however, results can be unpredictable.[32,56,57] Using standard harvesting and processing techniques, fat can be placed along the angle and body to augment its width. Blunt cannulas are inserted lateral to the mental foramen and passed along the mandible in a supraperiosteal plane. Small aliquots are placed in a retrograde and fanning approach to increase viability of the fat placed.

Genioplasty

The primary approach for masculinizing the chin consists of placement of alloplastic implants (silicone or Medpor). Implant insertion will aid in accentuating the width and projection of the chin, but cannot adequately increase vertical height. Using a submental approach, an incision is placed 2 mm behind the submental crease. After dissection to the mentalis muscle, this is elevated with or without the periosteum, with care taken not to injure the mental nerves. Implants are placed subperiosteal laterally and supraperiosteal centrally to minimize erosion. Monocortical screw fixation secures the implants to the lower jaw. The mentalis is reapproximated and soft tissue resuspended. Implants also can be inserted intraorally through a similar approach, as described later in this article, for sliding genioplasty, but the soft tissue must be stripped from the lower border of the mandible for placement of the implant. Fixation and closure are similar to mandibular implant placement, as described previously. Sliding genioplasty provides more options and flexibility for contouring the chin.

When sliding genioplasty is performed with the mandible angle augmentation, the incision described in that section can be used. If performed in isolation, a labial sulcus incision with a wide cuff of mucosa and cuff of mentalis is performed. Dissection of the anterior mandible is performed in a subperiosteal plane, with care taken to avoid the mental nerves. The lower border is stripped of its soft tissue attachments. Once exposed, a line 5 mm below the mental nerves bilaterally is marked. A reciprocating saw is used to make the initial cut for the osteotomy and it is completed with an osteotome. An oscillating saw is then used to open the central portion of the bone in the midline to allow for widening of the chin with or without an interposition bone graft or hydroxyapatite granules mixed with the patient's blood. The bony segments are fixed temporarily with wires if needed. The segments are advanced a predetermined amount for vertical augmentation and fixated with plates and screws. Once stable, the incisions are irrigated and closed in layers with Vicryl to resuspend the mentalis, then either Vicryl or Chromic to close the mucosa in a horizontal mattress fashion.

A less invasive approach involves fat transfer along the chin to increase width and projection of the lower face; however, results can be unpredictable.[32,56,57] Using standard harvesting and processing techniques, fat can be placed along the chin to augment its width. Blunt cannulas are inserted at the mental crease, chin apex, anterior chin, submental chin, and pre-jowl sulcus, and passed along the chin in a supraperiosteal plane. Small aliquots are placed in a retrograde and fanning approach to increase viability of the fat placed.

POSTOPERATIVE CARE

Typically when performed as a full-facial gender-affirming procedure, then patients are admitted to the hospital for overnight monitoring. If performed in isolation, then lower jaw contouring can be done as an outpatient procedure. If done as an outpatient, then follow-up in 1 to 2 days postoperatively is needed to ensure the patient is progressing appropriately (**Fig. 4**).

Most incisions will be placed within the mouth and closed with absorbable suture, so appropriate oral hygiene is needed. In most cases, this consists of antiseptic mouthwash (chlorhexidine gluconate) 3 times a day for 1 week (longer use may cause discoloration of teeth). Gentle brushing of teeth and rinsing with water or saline should be done after each meal. Patients are maintained on oral antibiotics for 1 week. A soft diet can be started after surgery and should continue for 4 weeks. Icing of the face and use of facial compression garments are used. Head of bed elevation is continued as much as possible to reduce swelling that will continue for weeks to months after surgery. Numbness of the lower lips and chin as a result of mental nerve neuropraxia is expected and generally resolves after 4 weeks, but can persist for up to a year. Normal activity restrictions and wound care of extraoral incisions are applied.

If a bone graft was harvested, then wound care to these incisions will be needed. Typically, iliac crest bone harvest does not warrant specific therapies. If fat grafting was used, then a compression garment is placed on the torso after surgery. This is continued for 2 weeks as much as possible, and then weaned over the next 4 weeks.

COMPLICATIONS AND OTHER PROCEDURES

As with any craniofacial procedures, there are inherent risks with modification of the facial bones. Specifically, in relation to the lower jaw, risks include infection (including implant, soft tissue, and osteomyelitis), wound dehiscence with exposure of underlying bony architecture, mental nerve injury or neuropraxia, inferior alveolar nerve injury, tooth root injury, nonunion of osteotomy sites, resorption of bone, mentalis muscle dysfunction, salivary fistulas, and iatrogenic injury to nearby structures. Most of these can be treated nonoperatively. Various studies have reported minimal to no surgical complications from lower jaw contouring for gender-affirming surgery.[31,33,34,52,58]

After modification of the craniofacial skeleton, changes to the soft tissue of the face may

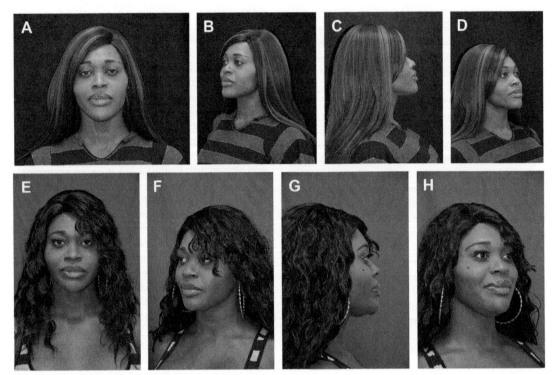

Fig. 4. Gender-affirming feminization. (*A–D*) Preoperative and (*E–H*) 6-month postoperative after genioplasty, mandibular angle and body reduction, and thyroid cartilage reduction.

occur. Modification with injectables, including neurotoxins, fillers, or fat grafting, may be useful.[64] Other soft tissue procedures, like submental and neck liposuction or a facelift, may be needed to adequately address underlying soft tissue anomalies. In particular, patients older than 40 (and those with inherent laxity in their skin) should be advised preoperatively that there is a possibility of needing a facelift or necklift after significant bony reduction of the chin and mandible.

OUTCOMES

Data on outcomes of facial gender-affirming surgery report few complications.[11] Patient-reported outcomes are sparse in current literature on facial gender-affirming surgery, with most studies that report these data using nonvalidated instruments.[11] One group has validated an instrument that has been used to assess retrospective quality-of-life outcomes in facial feminization surgery. Results show that transgender women had significantly diminished mental health quality of life compared with the non-transgender population, but this was significantly improved after facial feminization or gender-affirming surgery.[59] This instrument was used in another retrospective study that showed a high "facial feminization outcome

score," but was not compared with a standardized group.[42] A prospective study on outcomes of facial feminization has supported the results from this previous research and these data are currently being evaluated for long-term outcomes.[60] Further use of validated instruments in the assessment of outcomes for gender-affirming surgery is needed, along with input from community stakeholders among the transgender and gender nonbinary community on the development of these instruments, and this will be invaluable in future research in this field.[5,7,61–63]

SUMMARY

Lower jaw recontouring for facial gender-affirming surgery offers safe and effective means to masculinize or feminize the face. Shared decision-making between the physician and patient will allow for appropriate adjustments to portray the patient's true gender. Reported complications are minimal, but more robust research is needed, especially related to patient-reported outcomes. Our transgender and gender nonbinary patients deserve quality health care, and surgeons should seek to deliver that care through continued collaborations and multidisciplinary approaches.

REFERENCES

1. Coleman E, Bockting W, Botzer M, et al. Standards of care for the health of transsexual, transgender, and gender-nonconforming people, version 7. International Journal of Transgenderism 2019;13(4): 165–232.
2. Berli JU, Knudson G, Fraser L, et al. What surgeons need to know about gender confirmation surgery when providing care for transgender individuals: a review. JAMA Surg 2017;152(4):394–400.
3. Dhejne C, Lichtenstein P, Boman M, et al. Long-term follow-up of transsexual persons undergoing sex reassignment surgery: cohort study in Sweden. PLoS One 2011;6(2):e16885.
4. Ludwig DC, Morrison SD. Should dental care make a transition? J Am Dent Assoc 2018;149(2):79–80.
5. Massie JP, Morrison SD, Smith JR, et al. Patient-reported outcomes in gender confirming surgery. Plast Reconstr Surg 2017;140(1):236e–7e.
6. Morrison SD, Chen ML, Crane CN. An overview of female-to-male gender-confirming surgery. Nat Rev Urol 2017;14(8):486–500.
7. Morrison SD, Crowe CS, Wilson SC. Consistent quality of life outcome measures are needed for facial feminization surgery. J Craniofac Surg 2017;28(3): 851–2.
8. Morrison SD, Perez MG, Nedelman M, et al. Current state of female-to-male gender confirming surgery. Curr Sex Health Rep 2015;7:38–48.
9. Ascha M, Massie JP, Morrison SD, et al. Outcomes of single stage phalloplasty by pedicled anterolateral thigh flap versus radial forearm free flap in gender confirming surgery. J Urol 2018;199(1):206–14.
10. Morrison SD, Satterwhite T, Grant DW, et al. Long-term outcomes of rectosigmoid neocolporrhaphy in male-to-female gender reassignment surgery. Plast Reconstr Surg 2015;136(2):386–94.
11. Morrison SD, Vyas KS, Motakef S, et al. Facial feminization: systematic review of the literature. Plast Reconstr Surg 2016;137(6):1759–70.
12. Remington AC, Morrison SD, Massie JP, et al. Outcomes after phalloplasty: do transgender patients and multiple urethral procedures carry a higher rate of complication? Plast Reconstr Surg 2018; 141(2):220e–9e.
13. Massie JP, Morrison SD, Wilson SC, et al. Phalloplasty with urethral lengthening: addition of a vascularized bulbospongiosus flap from vaginectomy reduces postoperative urethral complications. Plast Reconstr Surg 2017;140(4):551e–8e.
14. Chaiet SR, Morrison SD, Streed CG Jr. Gender confirmation surgery and terminology in transgender health. JAMA Surg 2017;152(11):1089–90.
15. Massie JP, Streed CG Jr, Neira PM, et al. Terminology in transgender patient care. Plast Reconstr Surg 2018;141(2):317e–8e.
16. Canner JK, Harfouch O, Kodadek LM, et al. Temporal trends in gender-affirming surgery among transgender patients in the United States. JAMA Surg 2018;153(7):609–16.
17. Winter S, Diamond M, Green J, et al. Transgender people: health at the margins of society. Lancet 2016;388(10042):390–400.
18. Dubin SN, Nolan IT, Streed CG Jr, et al. Transgender healthcare: improving medical student and resident training and awareness. Adv Med Educ Pract 2018; 9:377–91.
19. Dy GW, Osbun NC, Morrison SD, et al. Exposure to and attitudes regarding transgender education among urology residents. J Sex Med 2016;13(10):1466–72.
20. Massenburg BB, Morrison SD, Rashidi V, et al. Educational exposure to transgender patient care in otolaryngology training. J Craniofac Surg 2018; 29(5):1252–7.
21. Morrison SD, Chong HJ, Dy GW, et al. Educational exposure to transgender patient care in plastic surgery training. Plast Reconstr Surg 2016;138(4): 944–53.
22. Morrison SD, Dy GW, Chong HJ, et al. Transgender-related education in plastic surgery and urology residency programs. J Grad Med Educ 2017;9(2): 178–83.
23. Morrison SD, Smith JR, Mandell SP. Are surgical residents prepared to care for transgender patients? JAMA Surg 2018;153(1):92–3.
24. Morrison SD, Wilson SC, Smith JR. Are we adequately preparing our trainees to care for transgender patients? J Grad Med Educ 2017;9(2):258.
25. Weissler JM, Chang BL, Carney MJ, et al. Gender-affirming surgery in persons with gender dysphoria. Plast Reconstr Surg 2018;141(3):388e–96e.
26. Morrison SD, Perez MG, Carter CK, et al. Pre- and post-operative care with associated intra-operative techniques for phalloplasty in female-to-male patients. Urol Nurs 2015;35(3):134–8.
27. Berli JU, Capitan L, Simon D, et al. Facial gender confirmation surgery—review of the literature and recommendations for version 8 of the WPATH standards of care. Int J Transgend 2017;18(3):264–70.
28. Wilson SC, Morrison SD, Anzai L, et al. Masculinizing top surgery: a systematic review of techniques and outcomes. Ann Plast Surg 2018;80(6):679–83.
29. Ousterhout DK. Feminization of the forehead: contour changing to improve female aesthetics. Plast Reconstr Surg 1987;79(5):701–13.
30. Ousterhout DK. Facial feminization surgery: a guide for the transgendered woman. Google eBook. San Francisco (CA): Addicus Books; 2010.
31. Ousterhout DK. Dr Paul Tessier and facial skeletal masculinization. Ann Plast Surg 2011;67(6):S10–5.
32. Altman K. Facial feminization surgery: current state of the art. Int J Oral Maxillofac Surg 2012;41(8): 885–94.

33. Becking AG, Tuinzing DB, Hage JJ, et al. Facial corrections in male to female transsexuals: a preliminary report on 16 patients. J Oral Maxillofac Surg 1996;54(4):413–8 [discussion: 419].

34. Becking AG, Tuinzing DB, Hage JJ, et al. Transgender feminization of the facial skeleton. Clin Plast Surg 2007;34(3):557–64.

35. Capitan L, Simon D, Kaye K, et al. Facial feminization surgery: the forehead. Surgical techniques and analysis of results. Plast Reconstr Surg 2014; 134(4):609–19.

36. Dempf R, Eckert AW. Contouring the forehead and rhinoplasty in the feminization of the face in male-to-female transsexuals. J Craniomaxillofac Surg 2010;38(6):416–22.

37. Deschamps-Braly JC, Sacher CL, Fick J, et al. First female-to-male facial confirmation surgery with description of a new procedure for masculinization of the thyroid cartilage (Adam's apple). Plast Reconstr Surg 2017;139(4):883e–7e.

38. Farkas LG, Hreczko TA, Kolar JC, et al. Vertical and horizontal proportions of the face in young adult North American Caucasians: revision of neoclassical canons. Plast Reconstr Surg 1985;75(3):328–38.

39. Habal MB. Aesthetics of feminizing the male face by craniofacial contouring of the facial bones. Aesthetic Plast Surg 1990;14(2):143–50.

40. Hage JJ, Becking AG, de Graaf FH, et al. Gender-confirming facial surgery: considerations on the masculinity and femininity of faces. Plast Reconstr Surg 1997;99(7):1799–807.

41. Hage JJ, Vossen M, Becking AG. Rhinoplasty as part of gender-confirming surgery in male transsexuals: basic considerations and clinical experience. Ann Plast Surg 1997;39(3):266–71.

42. Raffaini M, Magri AS, Agostini T. Full facial feminization surgery: patient satisfaction assessment based on 180 procedures involving 33 consecutive patients. Plast Reconstr Surg 2016;137(2):438–48.

43. Spiegel JH. Challenges in care of the transgender patient seeking facial feminization surgery. Facial Plast Surg Clin North Am 2008;16(2):233–8, viii.

44. Spiegel JH. Facial determinants of female gender and feminizing forehead cranioplasty. Laryngoscope 2011;121(2):250–61.

45. Cho DY, Massie JP, Morrison SD. Ethnic considerations for rhinoplasty in facial feminization. JAMA Facial Plast Surg 2017;19(3):243.

46. Lee SW, Ahn SH. Angloplasty revision: importance of genioplasty for narrowing of the lower face. Plast Reconstr Surg 2013;132(2):435–42.

47. Lundgren TK, Farnebo F. Midface osteotomies for feminization of the facial skeleton. Plast Reconstr Surg Glob Open 2017;5(1):e1210.

48. Bellinga RJ, Capitan L, Simon D, et al. Technical and clinical considerations for facial feminization surgery with rhinoplasty and related procedures. JAMA Facial Plast Surg 2017;19(3):175–81.

49. Capitan L, Simon D, Meyer T, et al. Facial feminization surgery: simultaneous hair transplant during forehead reconstruction. Plast Reconstr Surg 2017; 139(3):573–84.

50. Cho SW, Jin HR. Feminization of the forehead in a transgender: frontal sinus reshaping combined with brow lift and hairline lowering. Aesthetic Plast Surg 2012;36(5):1207–10.

51. Hoenig JF. Frontal bone remodeling for gender reassignment of the male forehead: a gender-reassignment surgery. Aesthetic Plast Surg 2011; 35(6):1043–9.

52. Ousterhout DK. Feminization of the chin: a review of 485 consecutive cases, vol. 10. Bologna (Italy): Medimond International Proceedings; 2003.

53. Sayegh F, Ludwig DC, Ascha M, et al. Facial masculinization surgery and its role in the treatment of gender dysphoria. J Craniofac Surg, in press.

54. Li J, Hsu Y, Khadka A, et al. Surgical designs and techniques for mandibular contouring based on categorisation of square face with low gonial angle in Orientals. J Plast Reconstr Aesthet Surg 2012; 65(1):e1–8.

55. Yaremchuk MJ, Chen YC. Enlarging the deficient mandible. Aesthet Surg J 2007;27(5):539–50.

56. Coleman SR. Facial augmentation with structural fat grafting. Clin Plast Surg 2006;33(4):567–77.

57. Coleman SR. Structural fat grafting: more than a permanent filler. Plast Reconstr Surg 2006;118(3 Suppl):108S–20S.

58. Shams MG, Motamedi MH. Case report: feminizing the male face. Eplasty 2009;9:e2.

59. Ainsworth TA, Spiegel JH. Quality of life of individuals with and without facial feminization surgery or gender reassignment surgery. Qual Life Res 2010; 19(7):1019–24.

60. Satterwhite T, Morrison SD, Ludwig DC, et al. Prospective quality of life outcomes after facial feminization surgery. Plast Reconstr Surg Glob Open 2017;5(9 Suppl):204–5.

61. Andreasson M, Georgas K, Elander A, et al. Patient-reported outcome measures used in gender confirmation surgery: a systematic review. Plast Reconstr Surg 2018;141(4):1026–39.

62. Morrison SD, Crowe CS, Rashidi V, et al. Beyond phonosurgery: considerations for patient-reported outcomes and speech therapy in transgender vocal feminization. Otolaryngol Head Neck Surg 2017; 157(2):349.

63. Morrison SD, Massie JP, Crowe CS, et al. Patient-reported outcomes needed for chest masculinization. Ann Plast Surg 2018;80(1):90–1.

64. Ascha M, Swanson MA, Massie JP, et al. Nonsurgical management of facial masculinization and feminization. Aesthet Surg J, in press.

Feminization of the Chin
Genioplasty Using Osteotomies

Jordan Deschamps-Braly, MD, FACS

KEYWORDS

- Sliding genioplasty • Chin feminization • Osseous genioplasty • Facial feminization surgery • FFS
- Facial gender confirmation surgery

KEY POINTS

- Male and female chins have markedly different characteristics, so chin reshaping is an important part of facial feminization surgery.
- Chin reshaping can change the chin's width, height, and contour, as well as correcting chins that are too prominent, recessed, or asymmetrical.
- The sliding osseous genioplasty is the most effective approach for creating a chin with a dramatically different female shape.
- Keeping 6 mm or more below the inferior border of the mental nerve canal during osteotomies performed in sliding genioplasty greatly reduces any risk of injury to the nerve.
- Virtual techniques can be used for each genioplasty to precisely plan each surgery to achieve the best aesthetic results and ensure safety.

INTRODUCTION

Chin reshaping is often a crucial part of facial feminization, because the chin plays such a large part in gender recognition. Men's chins are taller, wider, and often more projected than women's chins, which tend to have a softer, more tapered or oval appearance. Although the differences may seem subtle or inconsequential to an untrained observer, reducing the height of a chin by what amounts to millimeters can make a tremendous difference in the appearance of a male-to-female (MTF) transgender patient.

Because the chin is such an identifiable marker of gender, it needs to be altered in almost all feminization procedures to achieve the most aesthetic and feminine effects. We have performed facial feminization (FFS) on hundreds of transgender patients, and my associate, Douglas Ousterhout, has performed similar surgeries on close to 1500 patients. Between us, we found sliding genioplasty to be beneficial in all but a handful of patients who presented to our clinic. In fact, close to 99% of transgender patients will need to have their chins reshaped during facial feminization.

A male chin is on average approximately 20% taller than a female chin, and the male chin is also wider, with paired prominences that add to its square appearance. Besides changing the chin's width, height, and contour, a surgeon can refashion the face to correct chins that are too prominent, too recessed, or asymmetrical during FFS. The "sliding," or more appropriately called "osseous," genioplasty is the preferred and only effective approach for safely creating a more feminine shape (**Fig. 1**).

CONTENT

The sliding or osseous genioplasty is used to modify the chin by sectioning the chin and removing and or repositioning segments of the

Disclosure Statement: The author has no conflicts of interest or financial relationships that would influence our recommendations.
Deschamps-Braly Clinic of Plastic & Craniofacial Surgery, 360 Post Street, Suite 901, San Francisco, CA 94108, USA
E-mail address: info@deschamps-braly.com

Facial Plast Surg Clin N Am 27 (2019) 243–250
https://doi.org/10.1016/j.fsc.2019.01.002

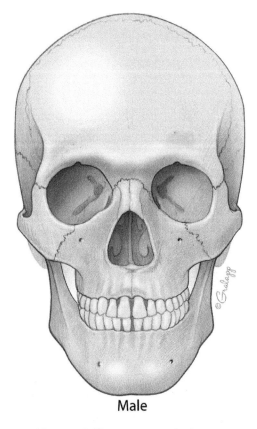

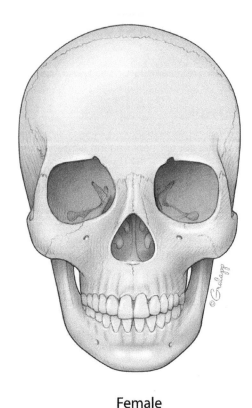

Male

Female

The male skull is more rectangular, has a vertically longer chin, and a wider, fuller jaw.

The female skull is more oval, has a vertically
shorter chin, and a more pointed chin.

Fig. 1. Comparison of the male versus the female chin. (Illustration ©2018 Chris Gralapp.)

bone and is thus the most effective approach for creating a female chin. By contrast, chin implants make the chin larger in one dimension or another, and, therefore, are counterproductive for most MTF transgender patients. Surface contouring by simple burring the "excess" bone is also unsatisfactory because it does not change the chin's prominence or height appreciably. To be successful in burring the excess bone, the amount of bone removed would need to be so large that the cancellous bone would be totally exposed. This would result in contour irregularities—a truly undesirable complication.

The first detailed review on feminization of the chin with 485 cases was published by my associate, Douglas Ousterhout, MD, DDS, FACS, in 2003.[1] Genioplasty was first described by Otto Hofer[2] in 1942, who published a description of a sliding advancement genioplasty performed on a cadaver via an external approach. Gillies and Millard[3] published the first scientific report of a genioplasty on a living patient in 1957, performed with an extraoral approach. The first modern osseous genioplasties were performed for microgenia after

it became understood that placement of bone grafts on the anterior surface of the chin tended to resorb with recurrence of the original deformity.

Trauner and Obwegeser[4] and Converse and Wood-Smith[5] later described sliding advancement genioplasties performed with an intraoral approach, published respectively in 1957 and 1964. It was not until the 1970s and 1980s, however, that the first descriptions of chin height reductions with wedge ostectomy were published by Hohl and Epker (1976)[6] and McBride and Bell (1980).[7]

In 1987, Wolfe[8] fully described methods for altering the vertical dimensions of the chin by shortening or lengthening it. In his report, Wolfe[8] noted that the results of chin lengthening had improved with the use of fixation by small plates. The technique described by Wolfe[8] for shortening the chin involved moving bone above the lower border of the symphysis, while preserving the muscular attachments to the lower border. The bone was then reattached to the remaining upper mandibular segment.[7,8] The methods described by Wolfe[8] have now been modified so that a

T-osteotomy of the chin is used to achieve vertical height or width reduction in FFS, and less commonly, advancement or setback.

Wolfe[8] noted in his 1987 paper that the extent of chin shortening could be limited by the position of the mental nerve. In fact, mental nerve injuries have long been a concern with sliding genioplasties, although the true incidence of these injuries has never been adequately documented. Yet in 1996, Ousterhout[9] reported on a prospective case series in which a method was used to successfully avoid mental nerve injuries.

Ousterhout's technique was based on an anatomic and radiographic study published in 1992,[10] which showed that there were no cases in which the mental nerve's course put it more than 5.5 mm below the inferior border of the mental foramen. Thus, all 50 osteotomies that were performed as part of Ousterhout's prospective case series were at least 6 mm below the inferior border of the mental nerve canal.

The results of Ousterhout's study[9] revealed that there were no mental nerve injuries among the patients who were part of the 50 prospective case cases. Ousterhout[9] then compared these results with those of his preceding 50 cases in which the distance of the osteotomy from the mental nerve was not recorded. Among these patients there were 3 permanent injuries:

- One bilateral complete numbness
- One unilateral complete numbness
- One unilateral partial numbness

In the 1992 study published in the *Journal of Craniofacial Surgery*, Ritter and colleagues[10] found that the course of the inferior alveolar neurovascular canal could be highly variable. In fact, the distance between the inferior border of the mandible to the lowest point in the inferior alveolar canal ranged from 2 to 11 mm in 52 cases assessed with radiographs. The position of the mental foramen also varied, ranging from 6 to 21 mm above the caudal border of the mandible in these cases; yet, the lowest point in the course of the nerve was always less than 6 mm.

The study suggested that the mental foramen was a useful landmark for the anterior intramandibular course of the inferior alveolar nerve. Low mental foramens in general correlated with low-lying nerves in the case series. The study supported the necessity of visually identifying the mental foramen with radiographs before sliding genioplasty, and performing the osteotomy at a minimum of 6 mm below the inferior margin of the mental foramen to avoid nerve injury.

"For many plastic surgeons, the idea of working with bone seems unfathomable, far too complicated and dangerous, and beyond the scope of their practice," Dr Ousterhout[9] wrote in his 1996 article. Thus, many plastic surgeons prefer to fix a retruded chin with an implant. Yet this is a relatively blind procedure and may result in mental nerve injuries from the procedure itself or the implants. Experience with implants has improved over time; however, problems still exist. Implant malposition is one of the most common things we see when problems with implants arise. In addition to an unfavorable appearance, I have personally seen erosion of malpositioned implants through the outer table of bone that resulted in the following:

- Loss of all 4 lower incisors
- Implant malposition that caused mental nerve paresthesias
- Capsules around the nerve causing something approximating mentalis strain

Other issues with implants are less common.

It cannot be said that osseous genioplasty is without some risk of complications; however, feminizing a chin, reducing the height of the chin, setting back a prominent chin, and correcting asymmetries cannot be performed with an implant. They require bony facial contouring procedures. Therefore, learning to perform these procedures well is imperative. Maintaining 6 mm or more below the inferior border of the mental nerve canal during sliding genioplasty cannot always rule out an injury to the nerve, but it greatly reduces the risk of such damage.

Before performing any genioplasty, we obtain a Panorex radiograph and a posterior to anterior and lateral cephalograms. In addition, I obtain a computed tomography (CT) scan of the patient's facial bones as well as 3D-dimensional scans of the teeth. Taken together along with good clinical photographs, these studies help to determine precisely what must be done during the sliding genioplasty.

The cephalometric measurements of each patient will be evaluated against various published male and female standards. The radiographs and CT scan are also used to mark the path of the inferior alveolar nerve along the lower border of the mandible and the precise position of the exit of the right and left mental nerves. It's also crucial to evaluate the relationship of the patient's chin to her facial configuration, especially the profile. Although the front and back positions of the chin vary tremendously in attractive people, they are always in balance with other facial areas. Published norms are a useful guideline, but one also needs the ability to visualize a pleasing profile for the patient and to determine which movements of the chin can approximate the intended shape and profile.

We use these measurements because they are necessary, but we also keep beauty and aesthetics in mind while developing our surgical plans. Because we are trying to achieve precise facial proportions, changes of only a few millimeters to the chin can make a big difference in feminizing the face. We have taken the chin height down as little as 2 mm and as much as 19 mm, although the amount removed varies from person to person.[11]

We also occasionally use virtual planning techniques to plan genioplasties. CT scans help us establish the guidelines for each genioplasty to achieve the most aesthetic and feminine results. With virtual planning, we can produce surgical guides that can ensure that the results we planned using CT scans are translated into real life. Virtual planning is not used in every case. Yet if certain details of the case call for it, the additional expense incurred in generating the guides and trying the surgery first in a virtual environment can be worth it.[11]

During the procedure, we work through incisions placed inside the mouth to avoid externally visible scars. The initial incision is made in the mobile gingiva, usually from the first molar on each side, which exposes the entire chin, including the mental nerves near the first and second bicuspid teeth root tips. We then do some basic contouring to remove any paired prominences that may be present. From there, we reduce height by first removing a horizontal piece of jawbone and then decrease width by cutting out a vertical segment. More often than not, these 2 maneuvers are performed simultaneously by removing a "T"-shaped piece of bone (**Fig. 2**). The remaining bone is then slid into place before securing it with a central titanium plate and screws. It is important to understand that ostectomy of the inferior border of the chin should be avoided. This creates a sharp edge that is palpable and has a high risk for disturbing the insertions of the genioglossus and anterior belly digastric muscles. This predisposes the patient to loss of cross-sectional airway volume.

Segmentation of the chin also requires additional placement of osteosynthesis plates laterally to stabilize the lateral chin segments. In a final step, we contour any edges that may be palpated due to the osteotomy. Although I use preoperative radiographs as a guide to excise bone for width reduction, I make the final decision about how much bone to remove and how much to contour the lateral prominences in the operating room.

As with jaw tapering, one of the most limiting factors to any chin surgery, particularly width reduction, is the basic shape of the dental arch. Whether it is tapered, oval, or square, the dental arch houses the roots of the teeth and mental

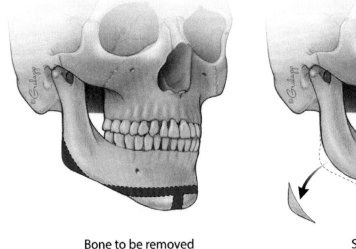

Bone to be removed

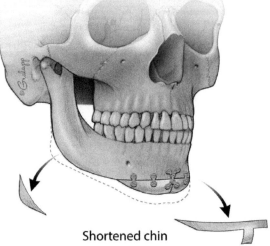

Shortened chin

Fig. 2. T-osteotomy of the chin with vertical and horizontal height reduction. (Illustration ©2018 Chris Gralapp.)

nerve, and all must be protected during surgery. This ensures safety, while we endeavor to make the face aesthetically pleasing and attractive.

Although the chin height is excessive in most transgender individuals, approximately 2% of patients need their chin heights increased. In these sliding genioplasties and osteotomies, we reposition the lower segment downward after the bone is cut horizontally. This creates space for new bone growth.

The segments are then stabilized with plates and screws. To help support the area temporarily, we insert a paste made from the patient's own blood. In addition, we insert the bone filler hydroxyapatite, made of sterile processed coral, and Avitene into the space, which provides excellent support until the bone develops.

Advancing a receding chin also can have a dramatic effect on anyone's face, particularly an MTF individual. Moving the chin forward as little as 3.2 mm or as much as 15.9 mm can markedly improve the patient's profile and appearance, while making the neck appear tighter and more attractive. To advance the chin, we make a horizontal cut in the lower mandible jaw and reduce the vertical excess. The inferior or lower portion of the bone is then slid forward and anchored in place with stabilizing titanium plates.

If a patient needs an advance that measures more than 10 mm, she is cautioned to wear a chin-strap for 6 weeks after surgery until the bone is completely healed. The length and cantilever-type projection of such chin advancements are so far forward that every movement of the genio-hyoids will pull the chin downward. The chinstrap has been very successful in preventing a relapse or a downward rotation of the prominent chin in our practice.

With an advancement of more than 6.4 mm, patients can experience an unattractive deepening of the sublabial sulcus. However, this can be addressed during the surgery. We treat it by placing a small amount of hydroxyapatite paste into the area as filler (**Figs. 3** and **4**).

The plates we use during genioplasties result in rigid fixation of the chin and along with maintaining some periosteal attachments to the chin segments, reduce the likelihood of bone resorption. By using the sliding genioplasty, we can also affect much greater advancement than we could with implants. The sliding genioplasty also narrows the chin, rather than widening it during FFS (**Figs. 5** and **6**).

The sliding genioplasty technique also can be used to reduce a prominent chin. After the bone cuts, the lower segments are positioned posteriorly for better alignment with the remainder of

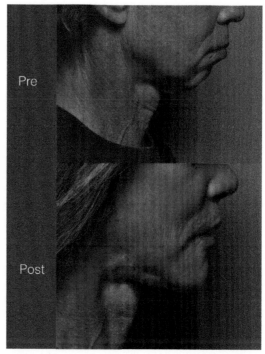

Fig. 3. Preoperative and postoperative large sliding genioplasty of 15 mm with use of hydroxyapatite granules. (*Courtesy of* Jordan Deschamps-Braly, MD, San Francisco, CA.)

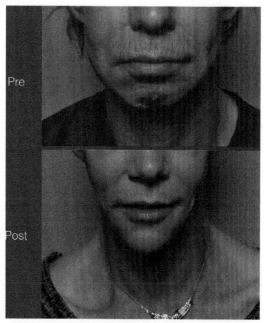

Fig. 4. Preoperative and postoperative large sliding genioplasty of 15 mm with use of hydroxyapatite granules. (*Courtesy of* Jordan Deschamps-Braly, MD, San Francisco, CA.)

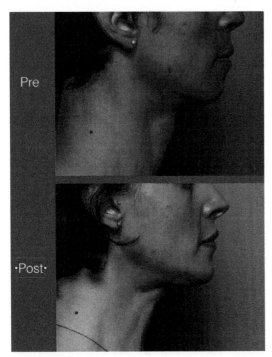

Fig. 5. Lateral view after chin osteotomy with vertical height reduction, narrowing, and advancement. (Courtesy of Jordan Deschamps-Braly, MD, San Francisco, CA.)

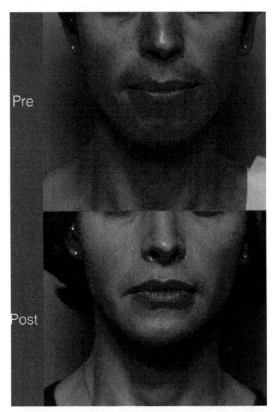

Fig. 6. Frontal view after chin osteotomy with vertical height reduction, narrowing, and advancement. (*Courtesy of* Jordan Deschamps-Braly, MD, San Francisco, CA.)

the features. Unfortunately, there is a limit to how much a surgeon can realistically set the bone back without affecting the submental-cervical angle. A setback of more than 5 mm usually causes skin and underlying tissue to accumulate between the chin and upper neck. If the bone is set back too far, we cannot achieve a truly clean, trim angle and the neck will appear fuller and more aged.

Correcting chin asymmetries can be accomplished with an osseous genioplasty technique as well. With this approach, we remove and asymmetrically reposition segments of bone to correct the imbalance. Usually the chin would be segmented, which allows differential movement of the segments. In performing these maneuvers, our aim is to improve the symmetry of the inferior border of the chin, the midline of the chin, and any asymmetry of the chin prominences. Chin asymmetry is not a common problem, but it occurs occasionally, and when it does, it must be corrected.

Over the years, we have revised many sliding genioplasties and chin implant operations performed by other surgeons. Patients have come to us because their previous surgeries did not result in a properly feminized chin or they had complications from the inserted implants. In

patients who have had implants and need further surgery, the implants can be removed, and a sliding genioplasty can be performed to correct any bone erosion and properly feminize the chin.

Most wrap-around chin implants of a large nature tend to remain stable; however, they make the chin appear significantly masculine. Narrower or smaller implants used in chin surgeries are more feminine, but they have a higher tendency to rotate, slide out of position, and erode into the bone. Also, implants rarely stay in the right position near the lower level of the chin bone. Instead, they migrate upward to a more stable but higher position. The result is a chin with an unusual abnormal rounded look in profile. Thus, surgery may be needed to remove the implants.

Revision cases after osseous genioplasties are very possible; however, it must be noted that previous hardware is often quite stubborn to remove. In many cases, the hardware must be cut using power tools. At times, this can leave residual metal in the bone. The reward for correcting such issues, however, is usually worth the effort when the final result becomes apparent.

After surgery, bone healing in the maxilla-mandibular skeleton is somewhat different from healing in the long bones of the body. On a radiograph, the line of the mandibular osteotomy may look like a "nonunion," or a fracture that has never healed completely. This appearance lasts almost indefinitely in some patients, but has no impact on the function of the jaws. On reoperating on patients who have had previous osteotomies, we find the bone is always healed despite these radiologic findings. For example, one patient of mine required removal of infected hardware 8 weeks after the initial surgery. The patient had already gone back overseas. The local radiologist was concerned that there was nonunion of the bone, thinking that the linear lucency on the radiograph meant it was not healed. I suggested that the line on the image was not worrisome and suggested that the plate should be immediately removed either locally or back in San Francisco. The bone was in fact healed on removal.

Since the introduction in the 1980s of internal plate and screw fixation, complications from sliding genioplasties have become increasingly rare. Yet they must be performed properly to prevent nerve injury and relapse. They also should be performed with an artistic eye and attention toward symmetry and proportion to avoid a safe but unpleasing result. Wound healing has never been a problem, and the number of infections we have had can be counted on one hand; yet after chin surgery, patients can experience some swelling beneath the lower jaw, particularly in the area just behind the chin osteotomy. The swelling seems to be caused by trapped blood under the periosteum. Usually this resolves, but if it does not, this osteophytic area may require another procedure to correct the excess fullness.

Thus far, I have not had to revise any chins because of relapse. My associate, D.K. Ousterhout, has revised 2 genioplasties because of relapse; the cause of these relapses, however, was not clearly evident. I have revised a few cases because of minor contour irregularities, or palpable hardware. In a few of Ousterhout's cases, the mental nerve was quite low, and the distal piece was shorter than usual. As a result, a small hourglass deformity occurred laterally. To remedy these cases, Ousterhout used 1 to 3 layers of 1-mm-thick MEDPOR, held together with 5 to 0 nylon suture along the side of the bone.[9] I have rarely found this necessary, and have often recommended extending the intraoral incisions sufficiently to perform some minor contouring of the mandible to blend the transition from the chin back along the body of the mandible. This has worked very well.

Many studies have assessed the safety of osseous genioplasty, and when appropriate precautions are taken, the mental nerve should remain undamaged and lip sensation remains intact. Usually some transient numbness occurs in the lips, but that resolves over the course of 2 years. Most often this transient numbness occurs when mandibular contouring is performed in conjunction with osteotomy of the chin. The reason for this is that the nerve must be retracted and manipulated to accomplish the contouring.

Since developing the procedure to avoid injuring the mental nerve, very few of our patients have experienced any permanent nerve damage. Some of my patients have described numbness in a very narrow vertical strip, approximately 3.2 mm wide down the middle of the lower lip and chin, sometimes involving the lower 2 or 4 incisor teeth.

After very large chin advancements (more than 12 mm), the patient also may perceive that her speech seems slurred when saying words that require the lips to touch during enunciation. Although the lower lip is moving perfectly, the patient may not feel it touching the upper lip because of temporary numbness. Although patients may perceive that they are not speaking properly, they actually have no speech problems, even with temporary numbness. This perception of "slurring" spontaneously resolves within 3 months.

In the past, major speech difficulties after a sliding genioplasty were a real, yet extremely rare, risk. The reason was some disturbance in the attachment of the genioglossus muscle. Occasionally a patient would complain of difficulty enunciating words after the surgeries. The situation occurred when there was a significant vertical reduction to the chin of 4.2 mm or more. We prevent this problem by stabilizing the base of the tongue muscle forward with a slowly degrading suture. Patients in our practice have not reported any major speech problems since we began using this approach years ago.

One of the great additional benefits of a feminizing sliding genioplasty is its effect on tooth show. Adult men have a large relative amount of lower tooth show when their mouths are slightly open. Women, however, show their upper teeth, rather than their lower teeth. Unfortunately, there is no good method for vertically lengthening the lower lip to give men a more feminized and reduced lower tooth display. However, the sliding genioplasty allows us to achieve that effect by reducing the underlying vertical height of the bony chin. This functionally allows for more coverage of the lower teeth by decreasing the ratio of bony height to soft tissue height. As a result, lower tooth show is markedly reduced and may even be eliminated after a properly completed feminizing genioplasty. The result is an overall feminizing effect on the lower jaw.

SUMMARY

To properly feminize the chin, it is necessary to understand the differences between male and female chins. To attempt to feminize the chin without considering the anatomic differences between men and women is like trying to steer a boat without a compass. Often, chin feminization entails reducing the height of the chin, narrowing the chin, and reducing its prominence. In some patients, there are also asymmetries or the chin is too retruded or long. Changing all these features of a chin and altering its position in FFS can best be accomplished with a single procedure.

Serious complications with these procedures are rare, and patient satisfaction is generally high. However, there are important cautions to consider. Mapping the course of the inferior alveolar nerve during preoperative planning is crucial in avoiding nerve injury during the sliding genioplasty. All anterior mandibular horizontal osteotomies also should be performed at least 6 mm below the inferior border of the mental foramen to protect the nerve. Patient education before surgery is also crucial, so that patients will have realistic expectations of the results that can be achieved and are informed about possible complications.

REFERENCES

1. Ousterhout DK. Feminization of the chin: a review of 485 consecutive cases, vol. 10. Bologna (Italy): Medimond International Proceedings; 2003.

2. Hofer O. Die operative Behandlung der alveolaren Retraktion des Unterkiefers und ihre Anwendungsmöglickkeit für Prognathie und Mikrogenie. Dtsch Zahn-Mund-Kieferheilkd 1942;9:121–32.

3. Gillies H, Millard DR. The principles and art of plastic surgery. Boston: Little, Brown; 1957. p. 361.

4. Trauner R, Obwegeser H. The surgical correction of mandibular prognathism and retrognathia with consideration of genioplasty. I. Surgical procedures to correct mandibular prognathism and reshaping of the chin. Oral Surg Oral Med Oral Pathol 1957;10: 677–89.

5. Converse JM, Wood-Smith D. Horizontal osteotomy of the mandible. Plast Reconstr Surg 1964; 34:464.

6. Hohl TH, Epker BN. Macrogenia: a study of treatment results, with surgical recommendations. Oral Surg Oral Med Oral Pathol 1976;41(5):545–67.

7. McBride KL, Bell WH. Chin surgery. In: Bell WH, Proffitt WR, White RP, editors. Surgical correction of dentofacial deformities, vol. II. Philadelphia: Saunders; 1980. p. 1238–40.

8. Wolfe SA. Shortening and lengthening the chin. J Craniomaxillofac Surg 1987;15(4):223–30.

9. Ousterhout DK. Sliding genioplasty, avoiding mental nerve injuries. J Craniofac Surg 1996;7(4): 297–8.

10. Ritter EF, Moelleken BR, Mathes SJ, et al. The course of the inferior alveolar neurovascular canal in relation to sliding genioplasty. J Craniofac Surg 1992;3(1): 20–4.

11. Ousterhout DK, Deschamps-Braly J. Feminization surgery: a guide for the transgendered woman. Omaha (NE): Addicus Books; 2010.

Gender-confirming Rhinoplasty

Jens Urs Berli, MD[a],*, Myriam Loyo, MD[b]

KEYWORDS

- Rhinoplasty • Transgender • Facial feminization surgery • Gender confirmation surgery
- Gender-affirming surgery

KEY POINTS

- Despite technical overlap, the care for patients seeking rhinoplasty for the indication of gender dysphoria vastly differs from that for the cisgender population.
- Rhinoplasty is often performed in combination with other facial gender-confirming surgeries. This article outlines important concepts that need to be taken into consideration.
- The facial gender mosaic concept is a useful tool to both assess patients and provide affirming care.

INTRODUCTION

Facial gender confirmation surgery (FGCS) encompasses a wide variety of surgical procedures, with the common goal of either feminizing or masculinizing the face. A vast majority of patients presenting for consultation are those seeking feminization procedures. Additionally, most facial plastic surgeons who are not routinely treating gender dysphoric patients are much more likely to see an isolated rhinoplasty consultation rather than a request for full facial feminization. Thus, this article focuses on feminizing rhinoplasty as it pertains to gender confirmation surgery. Different from other aspects of FGCS, the surgical basis of feminizing rhinoplasty is almost the same as for the cisgender population. Despite technical overlap, however, the management and care for patients seeking feminizing rhinoplasty for the indication of gender dysphoria vastly differs from that for the cisgender population. It is, therefore, important to understand these nuances to provide the best possible care. Most readers of this article are familiar with the general rhinoplasty literature and it is the

authors' hope that that this knowledge be augmented so that the experience of treating patients seeking feminizing rhinoplasty is rewarding for both patients and surgeons.

This review includes comments on gender norms and outlines considerations for the preoperative work-up and operative execution as well as a comprehensive literature review.

PREOPERATIVE MANAGEMENT

Successfully treating the severe experience of gender dysphoria is not just a question of technical skills and rhinoplasty expertise. It also requires sensitive and affirming care from the moment the patient calls the office but most importantly during the initial consultation. The overall experience to the transgender patient is of utmost importance.

Facial Gender Mosaic Concept

Even during an isolated rhinoplasty consultation, the authors strongly advocate that the surgeon focus on the entire facial appearance and let

Disclosure: None of the authors has any financial conflicts of interest.
[a] Division of Plastic Surgery, Department of General Surgery, Oregon Health & Science University, 3181 SW Sam Jackson Park Road, Mail Code L352A, Portland, OR 97201, USA; [b] Division of Facial Plastic and Reconstructive Surgery, Department of Otolaryngology–Head and Neck Surgery, Oregon Health & Science University, Center for Health and Healing, CH5E, 3303 Southwest Bond Avenue, Portland, OR 97201, USA
* Corresponding author.
E-mail address: jens.berli@gmail.com

Facial Plast Surg Clin N Am 27 (2019) 251–260
https://doi.org/10.1016/j.fsc.2019.01.003
1064-7406/19/© 2019 Elsevier Inc. All rights reserved.

patients point out aspects of their face that they perceive as affirming of their identified gender first. It is advised to avoid strong wording around masculine features and, unless specifically requested to, avoid pointing out those features. On the other hand, it is beneficial to point out the gender-affirming facial features that the patient may already have. The authors refer to this as the "facial gender mosaic" concept. Each face contains feminine and masculine traits. To start out by acknowledging and demonstrating the feminine aspects, the authors potentially assist patients in seeing these aspects for the first time. This not only helps build trust but also lays a foundation to see a patient's authentic female face. Bringing the discussion back to the nose at the end of the consultation and how the nose interacts with other discussed aspects of the face. To fruitfully engage in this conversation, the surgeon must also be informed on gender norms as well as ethnic considerations.

Patient Expectations

Patients seeking FGCS look for a face that is congruent with and affirming of their gender identity. Although this statement sounds simple, it only covers one aspect of the surgical plan: to achieve the opposite gender norm (discussed later). It does not address the version of the nose that is most congruent with patients' anatomy and genetics or patients' internal vision of themselves. Complicating this is that patients often have a negative self-image as it pertains to the face and may have avoided photographs and mirrors for years. In contrast, a cisgender patient often has specific concerns around nasal appearance. For

trans-identified patients, a frequently cited request is to make the nose "smaller" and "more sloped." It is, therefore, advised that the conversation around goals starts with the current anatomy and potentially involves photographs of female family members and of perceived ideals.

Setting expectations necessarily involves a thorough evaluation of the intricate anatomy of the nose with its innumerable variations. No single operative plan can be applied to all noses and myriad surgical maneuvers are necessary to successfully perform a feminizing rhinoplasty. On external examination, the skin quality deserves particular attention. Skin thickness and quality may limit the degree of nasal tip refinement that can be accomplished (**Fig. 1**). Exogenous estrogen can have marked effects on skin quality and it may be advised to await the full effect that usually sets in approximately 1 year to 2 years after initiation. The surgeon should discuss realistic expectations and define goals. Simulation software and imaging can assist in this discussion. A commonly heard prejudice is that the transgender patient population has a high degree of body dysmorphia; however, in the authors' experience, this has not been found true.

Functional Considerations as They Pertain to Facial Gender Confirmation

Analogous to rhinoplasties in cisgender patients, functional aspects leading to nasal obstruction need to be taken into consideration, including septal deviation, internal and external valves, and the inferior turbinates. Based on current literature, it can be assumed that there is a higher rate of obstructive sleep apnea in the trans-female

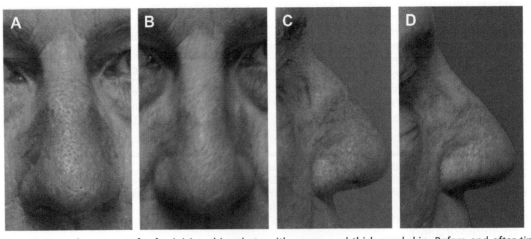

Fig. 1. Patient who presents for feminizing rhinoplasty with porous and thick nasal skin. Before and after tip refinement and dorsal hump reduction through an open approach. Patient did not want to have a slope. (A, C) Preoperative. (B, D) Postoperative. Result limited by thick skin envelope. (*Courtesy of* Dr Jens Berli.)

population compared with the cisgender female population; as such, this should be included in the preoperative discussion. Presence of obstructive sleep apnea may be a relative contraindication to combined jaw surgery and rhinoplasty.[1]

Fig. 2 shows a patient who presented for a secondary functional rhinoplasty due to persistent septal deviation and internal valve obstruction but also requesting feminization of the nasal tip.

Gender and Ethnic Differences in Nasal Anatomy

Before diving into the discussion of norms, it should be pointed out that ideals are subject to the times and culture lived in.(Fig. 3) There are gender norms that are likely to represent the binary ends of the gender spectrum. Dr Spiegel[2] makes the argument that it is beneficial to try to achieve these extremes because this may assist in decreasing the incidence of being misgendered. Going unrecognized in society as being the opposite gender assigned at birth is probably the most important outcome parameter of FGCS.

The authors agree with the spirit of decreasing cues that increase the probability of misgendering and also believe that patients should be directly involved in the decision because not everyone necessarily wants an appearance altered to match what a surgeon considers the binary end of the spectrum. For example, Fig. 4 shows a patient who had been recommended dorsal hump reduction and tip work during a feminizing FGCS consultation at a different office, but she preferred to have a straight dorsum and keep her rotation. Her rhinoplasty was performed to feminize her appearance and meet her specific goals.

Another critical consideration is ethnicity and cultural context. A patient with an indigenous American heritage may not want a sloped dorsum because it is not congruent with her ancestry; for this patient, a mild hump or straight nose may be more desirable. On the other hand, another patient of the same ethnic background may live in a different cultural context and desire to blend in with her surroundings, thereby having different goals for her appearance. Ethnic and cultural aspects should be part of the preoperative discussion.

Lastly, cultural trends should be considered within the context of longer-term goals. A patient

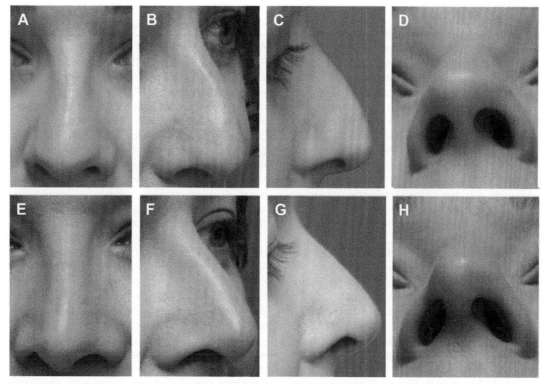

Fig. 2. Patient with status post–closed septorhinoplasty in the past with persistent deviated septum and internal valve obstruction. Functional revision and feminizing rhinoplasty performed through an open approach with component dorsal hump reduction, trapezoid spreader grafts with approximation of upper lateral cartilages, cephalic trim, tip sutures, alar rim, and columellar strut grafts. (A–D) are preoperative. (E–H) are postoperative. (Courtesy of Dr Jens Berli.)

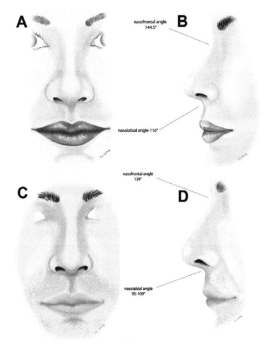

Fig. 3. Drawing of an example of a white gender norm. (*A, B*) are female gender normal. (*C, D*) are male gender normal. (*Courtesy of* Jens Berli and Jourdan Carboy.)

width of the nasal pyramid is wider in men than in women, with the dorsal aesthetic lines straight in the male ideal versus concave the female. The masculine nose is also more projected, with an average projection of 34 mm in men and 29.6 mm in women. Springer and colleagues[3] also noted the nasal tip rotation is decreased in men compared with women. Tanna and colleagues[4] report a nasolabial angle of approximately 95° to 100° in men and 100° to 110° in women. Decreasing nasal projection and increasing nasal tip rotation is a frequent goal of feminizing rhinoplasty. The degree of expected columellar show based on gender is a matter of debate. In the study by Springer and colleagues,[3] women had an increase columellar show compared with men. No such difference was seen in the Tanna and colleagues[4] study. The alar base width is another aspect that is markedly different. The Springer and colleagues[3] study cited a 4-mm difference in alar width between genders whereas men had a wider alar base. Lastly, they report length of the cutaneous upper lip is longer by 4 mm in men versus women. These differences lead to use of alar base reduction and subnasal lip lift during FCGS and feminizing rhinoplasty.

Financial and Psychosocial Aspects

As transgender people become more visible, FGCS has expanded. Third-party insurers and self-insurers, as well as some state insurance markets, are considering FGCS a covered benefit, rejecting the notion that FGCS is an aesthetic intervention. Even in this climate, FGCS remains costly and out of reach for many patients. Transgender people face numerous economic and health disparities, and understanding the psychosocial health of patients is an important consideration in planning for surgery.[5] Complicating social factors, such as financial hardship, unsafe home environments, unemployment, poverty, and even homelessness, can be present. The authors have encountered multiple patients who had previous self-inflicted nasal trauma with the hope to qualify for a posttraumatic rhinoplasty. Evaluation of a patient's psychosocial condition is, therefore, particularly important in these vulnerable patient populations. In particular, patients who have not yet transitioned socially should be encouraged to have a mental health professional at their side assisting them throughout the social transition period that may come with significant stressors.

It is incumbent on surgeons and their office staff to help patients understand if their insurance would cover the procedure.

may present early in her life and seek to be feminized as to the latest trends on social media, but later in life find she lost a facial uniqueness she now desires. These aspects should be part of an educated discussion with the patient.

To help guide this discussion, the authors find it helpful to ask patients to bring in photographs of female family members and perceived ideals.

Gender norms of the face are profoundly impacted by the advent of puberty. Once testosterone levels rise, the bony and cartilaginous framework of the face undergoes marked changes. Similarly, the soft tissue envelope experiences change with increase in porous diameter and dermal thickness.

The expansion of the frontal sinus in male puberty leads to a more acute nasofrontal (NF) angle. Springer and colleagues[3] published a photographic study evaluating the white gender norms as they pertain to nasal anatomy. They noted an optimal NF of 129° in men compared to 144.5° in women. This angle is not addressed adequately by rhinoplasty alone but requires frontal bone reduction (discussed later). The radix is also generally higher in men. The ideal feminine position cited by Springer and colleagues[3] is just above the pupil, whereas in men it is at the upper lid crease. Men in most Asian and some African races, however, have a radix that is lower. The

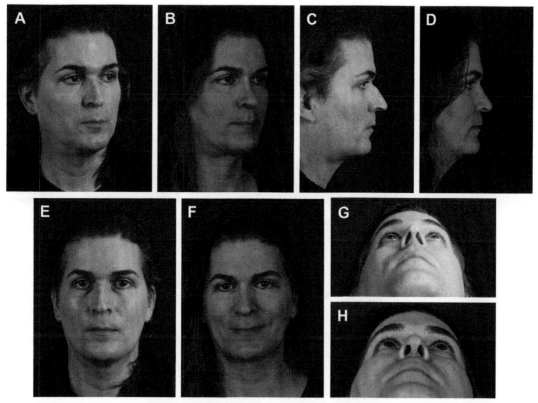

Fig. 4. A hump reduction with radix grafting was used to refine the nasal dorsum. Upper lateral cartilage turn-in flaps were used for the midvault. Projection of the nasal tip was decreased, and rotation was maintained per the patient's request. Cephalic turn-in flaps and alar rim graft were used. An alar base reduction was done to address alar flaring after decreasing projection. (*A, C, E,* and *G*) Preoperative. (*B, D, F,* and *G*) Postoperative. (*Courtesy of Dr Myriam Loyo.*)

Note on Gendered Language and Nonbinary Identity

A critical consideration of humane care for transgender identifying patients is respecting a patient's stated gender identity. For the novice to this field, this can be particularly challenging when confronted with patients who do not identify on the binary gender spectrum. In the authors' experience, nonbinary identified patients seeking gender surgery of the chest are almost exclusively female assigned at birth, whereas patients seeking FGCS predominantly are male assigned at birth. Patients should be asked for their preferred pronouns, and the surgeon and all office staff should ensure correct pronoun use. Misgendering by medical personnel has been cited as stressful and, in some cases, traumatic to patients, many of whom carry previous psychosocial trauma.[5,6] Although in-depth discussion of affirming language outside the scope of this article, it is recommended to access frequently updated resources because the language around this care is still

evolving. Finally, note that the use of "masculine/male" and "feminine/female" in this anatomic discussion follows gender norms based on gender assigned at birth.

FEMINIZING RHINOPLASTY—TECHNICAL CONSIDERATIONS
Dorsum/Radix

In the profile, the dorsal projection and slope are usually changed to a straight or slightly concave shape that assists in opening the NF angle. (**Figs. 4–6**) A useful guideline for nasal dorsum projection is to draw a line from the nasion to the ideal nasal tip position and have the dorsal projection be 1 mm to 2 mm posterior to this line. As discussed previously, ethnic variations may affect this and should be taken into consideration.

In the front view, reducing the width of the dorsal bridge is common, with the goal to have concave rather than straight dorsal aesthetic lines. The optimal width has been described as 75% to

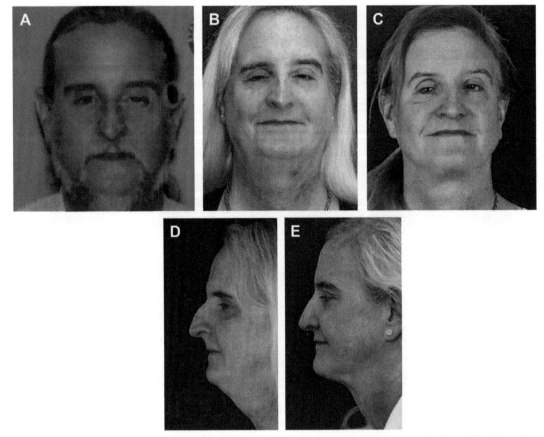

Fig. 5. The procedures performed included hairline lowering, forehead contouring, right browlift, rhinoplasty, and neck lift. The techniques used for rhinoplasty included a hump reduction and radix grafting for the nasal dorsum and tongue-in-groove to rotate and deproject the nose and cephalic turn in flaps to refine the nasal tip. (*A*) Prior to gender transition. (*B, D*) preoperative. (*C, E*) Postoperative. (*Courtesy of* Dr Myriam Loyo.)

80% of the alar base width in a female patient with normal alar base width.[7] With these goals in mind, it is common for feminizing rhinoplasty to include technical maneuvers, such as narrowing osteotomies, hump reductions, and radix grafting. Hage and colleagues[8] reported on 22 feminizing rhinoplasties where they used lateral and medial osteotomies in all cases and performed a hump reduction in slightly more than 50% of patients. The NF angle has been used by several investigators as an outcome measure that describes the changes in dorsal shape in feminization rhinoplasty. Nouraei and colleagues[9] from the United Kingdom describe an increase in NF angle from 142° to 151°. These investigators also increased the supratip angle from 2° to 13°. Similarly, Bellinga and colleagues[10] from Spain reported a change in the NF angle from 134° to 149° in their cohort, which includes 200 patients and is the largest cohort to date. In rhinoplasty cases of dorsal reduction, it is important to remember the

important function of spreader grafts to stabilize the shape of the dorsum and provide support to the internal nasal valve.

Tip Work

Modifying the nasal tip has been deemed the hardest part of rhinoplasty by many expert rhinoplasty surgeons because of delicate nature of the modifications. Nasal tip refinement is an almost universal goal of feminizing rhinoplasty. Understanding the tripod concept of the nose is essential in understanding how changes to 1 cartilage affect the overall 3-D structure of the nasal tip. Surgeons performing feminizing rhinoplasty need to successfully decrease nasal tip projection, increase rotation, and decrease width. Especially in feminizing rhinoplasty, this can be daunting because the tip often is severely overprotected and underrotated. Compared with cisnormative rhinoplasty, the feminizing rhinoplasty often necessitates

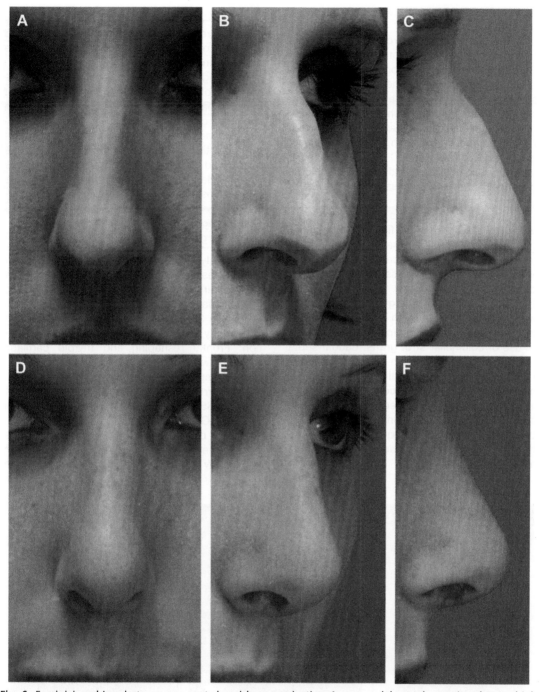

Fig. 6. Feminizing rhinoplasty: component dorsal hump reduction 4mm, caudal septal resection, low to high osteotomies bilateral, cephalic trim, LLC overlay, alar rim grafts, tip defining sutures, temporal-parietal fascia and diced cartilage dorsal onlay graft. Patient also had forehead reduction and browlift. (*Courtesy of* Jens Berli, MD.)

more aggressive techniques to not only normalize the projection within the natal gender norm but also transition it to the feminine spectrum. Nouraei and colleagues[9] reported changes in nasal tip rotation during feminizing rhinoplasty by reporting the nasolabial angle increase from 107° to 115°. Nouraei and colleagues[9] also reported that tip modifications were their only modification in approximately half of their cases (5 of 12 cases). Care should be taken when increasing nasal tip rotation to control tip projection and prevent an unnatural supra tip break.

Successfully decreasing projection of the nasal tip may require an interrupted strip technique with either overlay or resection of a portion of the lower lateral crura (LLC). When LLC are divided, asymmetric healing and scarring are concerns and meticulous operative technique is necessary. Refining the nasal tip considers the overall shape of the LLC and the position of the tip defining points. The shape of the LLC can be modified to flatten convex cartilages and reduce a bulbous tip as well as reduce excessively wide LLC by means of cephalic trim.

Nasal tip suture techniques and nasal tip grafts can be used to address the final nasal tip definition. When modifying the nasal tip, creating a stable construct and using cartilage grafting to restore nasal tip support is essential in preventing postoperative collapse. As part of the nasal tripod, the shape and strength of the columella should also be considered to prevent postoperative deviations and prevent tip ptosis considering the use of columellar strut grafts, caudal septal extension grafts, or tongue in groove techniques. In addition to the tripod cartilages, the final alar shape should be carefully considered, particularly in cases of dramatic reduction of the LLC width in which alar retraction could occur postoperatively. The authors frequently use alar rim grafts to prevent alar retraction and external valve collapse.

Alar Base

Alar base reduction is most commonly performed after the other structural changes to the nose have been completed. A useful guideline in considering alar base reduction is to compare the width of the ala to the intercanthal distance; if the alar base is wider, an alar base reduction should be considered. Alar flare that was not present preoperative can occur after deprojection of the nasal tip, and alar base reduction should be considered for these cases. Planning the incisions to camouflage the scars is extremely important to prevent unsightly scars (**Fig. 7**).

Combining Feminizing Rhinoplasty with Other Surgeries

Rhinoplasty is frequently combined with other procedures to achieve a feminization. A review of the literature confirms this and is reviewed here. Raffaini and colleagues[11] out of Italy reported on 33 FGCS patients who all underwent rhinoplasty, jaw contouring, and lip augmentation. Frontal reshaping and thyroid cartilage reduction were performed in 94% and 79% of patients, respectively. Similarly, Hage and colleagues[8] from the Netherlands reported that 21 (60%) of 35 patients had a rhinoplasty as part of another FGCS surgery. In the Bellinga and colleagues[10] case series, 75% of the 200 patients had forehead feminization in combination with rhinoplasty and only 2.5% of patients underwent

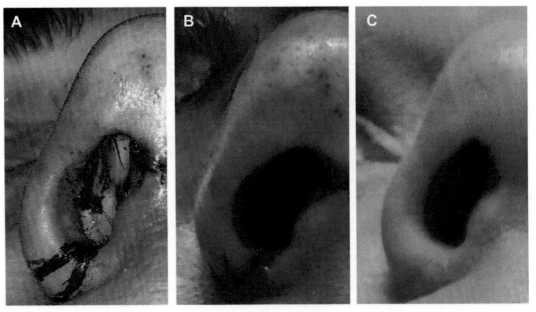

Fig. 7. Close-up view of alar base excision with the planned incisions to be hidden in the nasal sil. (*A*) Perioperative. (*B*) Immediately postoperative. (*Courtesy of* Dr Jens Berli.)

an isolated rhinoplasty. Because this team is specifically set up as a global destination for feminizing procedures, it can be postulated that providers in the United States will have a higher rate of requests for isolated rhinoplasty.

There are differences of opinion among surgeons regarding whether to combine rhinoplasty and a forehead feminization or perform the procedures separately. Raffaini and colleagues[11] advocated performing rhinoplasty first and delaying forehead contouring for 6 months when the jawline and nose are less swollen. In contrast, Bellinga and colleagues[10] frequently combine rhinoplasty and forehead contouring. The Bellinga and colleagues[10] study also exposes the nasal radix through the bicoronal approach and when necessary to reduce the radix. Both studies have published beautiful results that meet the goal of facial feminization. The authors agree with the Bellinga and colleagues[10] study, that improved exposure of the radix is possible when combining the forehead feminization and rhinoplasty. As for sequence during the surgery, the authors recommend performing the rhinoplasty last because the forehead flap can compress the nose.

When combining rhinoplasty with mandible and chin procedures, Bellinga and colleagues[10] recommend starting the surgery by using nasotracheal intubation for the mandibular procedures and subsequently exchanging the endotracheal tube to an oral tube to proceed with the rhinoplasty. In the authors' practice, forehead, mandibular, and nasal procedures are combined during the same procedure and the procedures performed with orotracheal intubation without exchanging tube position during surgery.

Lip lift procedures are intended to reduce the vertical height of the cutaneous upper lip, increase vermillion, and achieve upper incisor show. The literature and the authors' experience show that this can safely be performed during the same surgery (**Figs. 8 and 9**). Two groups have published on this combination of procedures with excellent results and no reported ischemic insults. Insalaco and Speigal[12] published a case series of 105 cases in which the transcolumellar incision was used for an open rhinoplasty approach and a separate incision was used for the lip lift. Bellinga and colleagues[10] reported 12% of their patients undergoing rhinoplasty also underwent a lip lift concomitantly (total 24 patients). In their series, the entire rhinoplasty is performed through a subnasal lip lift incision. Insalaco and Speigal[12] specifically comment on resecting skin from the columella during rhinoplasty in cases of significant nasal tip deprojection.[12] If alar base reduction is intended during surgery, placement of these incisions also should be considered. Delaying the lip lift until the alar reduction incision has healed is a reasonable consideration to prevent nostril stenosis and excessive scarring.

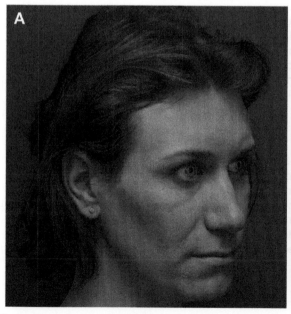
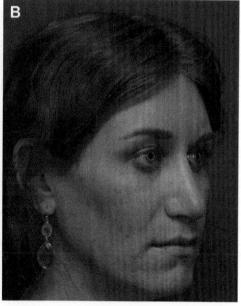

Fig. 8. The procedures performed included forehead contouring with sinus setback, tracheal shave, feminizing rhinoplasty, and lip lift. Incisions: columellar stair step and separate subnasal lip lift incision. (*A*) Preoperative. (*B*) Postoperative. (*Courtesy of* Dr Jens Berli.)

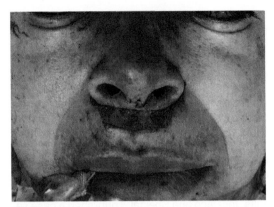

Fig. 9. Demonstration of the 2 separate incisions. (*Courtesy of* Dr Jens Berli.)

REVISIONS

Achieving patient satisfaction after rhinoplasty for gender confirmation involves a combination of meticulous technical maneuvers and open communication to discuss expectations and perceptions of femininity. In the cases series by Nouraei and colleagues,[9] several patients stated that their rhinoplasty was of the factors with the greatest impact in being perceived as female. The few case series that specify revision rates for feminizing rhinoplasties report rates and indications similar to larger cisgender rhinoplasty case series.[13] Hage and colleagues[8] reported that 18% of patients underwent revision after feminizing rhinoplasty (4 of 22 patients). In this case series, all patients reported a more feminine appearance. The largest case series of feminizing rhinoplasty is by Bellinga and colleagues[10] from Spain. In this case series, 4% of patients underwent revision (8 of the 200 patients). The reported indications for revision rhinoplasty were dorsal irregularities, unmet expectations of tip refinement, and chronic infection of the nasal tip.

SUMMARY

Surgeons offering feminizing rhinoplasty not only should be proficient with technical aspects of feminizing rhinoplasty but also have the necessary knowledge and compassion to provide affirming care. A comprehensive preoperative assessment and setting realistic expectations are crucial to successfully treating gender dysphoria associated with facial features.

ACKNOWLEDGMENTS

Seva Khambadkone, BS, for her help with editing the article. Kylie Blume, BS, MA, for her help with editing the article and submission process.

REFERENCES

1. Lin CM, Davidson TM, Ancoli-Israel S. Gender differences in obstructive sleep apnea and treatment implications. Sleep Med Rev 2008;12(6):481–96.
2. Spiegel JH. Rhinoplasty as a significant component of facial feminization and beautification. JAMA Facial Plast Surg 2017;19(3):181–2.
3. Springer IN, Zernial O, Nölke F, et al. Gender and nasal shape: measures for rhinoplasty. Plast Reconstr Surg 2008;121(2):629–37.
4. Tanna N, Nguyen KT, Ghavami A, et al. Evidence-based medicine: current practices in rhinoplasty. Plast Reconstr Surg 2018;141(1):137e–51e.
5. Grant JM, Mottet L, Tanis JE, et al. Injustice at every turn: a report of the national transgender discrimination survey. National Center for Transgender Equality; 2011.
6. Socías ME, Marshall BD, Arístegui I, et al. Factors associated with healthcare avoidance among transgender women in Argentina. Int J Equity Health 2014;13(1):81.
7. Papel ID, Frodel JL, Holt GR. Facial plastic and reconstructive surgery. Thieme; 2016.
8. Hage JJ, Vossen M, Becking AG. Rhinoplasty as part of gender-confirming surgery in male transsexuals: basic considerations and clinical experience. Ann Plast Surg 1997;39(3):266–71.
9. Nouraei SR, Randhawa P, Andrews PJ, et al. The role of nasal feminization rhinoplasty in male-to-female gender reassignment. Arch Facial Plast Surg 2007;9(5):318–20.
10. Bellinga RJ, Capitán L, Simon D, et al. Technical and clinical considerations for facial feminization surgery with rhinoplasty and related procedures. JAMA Facial Plast Surg 2017;19(3):175–81.
11. Raffaini M, Magri AS, Agostini T. Full facial feminization surgery: Patient satisfaction assessment based on 180 procedures involving 33 consecutive patients. Plast Reconstr Surg 2016;137(2):438–48.
12. Insalaco L, Spiegel JH. Safety of simultaneous lip-lift and open rhinoplasty. Jama Facial Plast Surg 2017; 19(2):160–1.
13. Guyuron B, Bokhari F. Patient satisfaction following rhinoplasty. Aesthetic Plast Surg 1996;20(2):153–7.

Lip Lift

Ara A. Salibian, MD, Rachel Bluebond-Langner, MD*

KEYWORDS

- Facial feminization • Lip lift • Gender-affirming surgery • Gender-confirmation surgery

KEY POINTS

- Gendering-affirming lip lifts must consider known aesthetic ideals of the female upper lip.
- Patient selection, preoperative education, and shared decision-making are key in minimizing complications and optimizing patient satisfaction.
- Patients' preoperative upper incisal show, alar base width, nasal sill prominence, skin tone and thickness, and vertical maxillary height must all be taken into consideration when planning lip lifts.
- The bullhorn-type subnasal lip lift is designed to achieve optimal lift along the entire upper lip (as afforded by alar base width) and hide scars at the nasal base under the nasal sill.

INTRODUCTION

Male and female faces have a multitude of different distinct features that create an overall masculine or feminine appearance. Facial feminization procedures have been designed to address several of these characteristics, primarily targeting the forehead, nose, and jawline.[1] The lips, however, are an aesthetic focal point of the lower face that have gender-specific features. The lip lift shortens the distance from the nasal base to the vermilion border using skin excision and tissue advancement. Although the procedure results in a subtle change, it can dramatically feminize the appearance of the lower face.

The indirect upper lip lift was first described for lip rejuvenation to treat senile upper lip ptosis and vermilion thinning.[2] The subnasal lift, or "bullhorn lip lift," uses a curved excision pattern along the nasal sill and alar creases to remove upper lip skin while hiding the scar along the nasal base, Multiple different variations of this procedure have been described.[3–7] The subnasal lip lift has been demonstrated to significantly decrease total upper lip and prolabium height, and increase vermilion height,[8] creating an upper lip that more closely resembles the described aesthetic ideals.[9]

These changes in upper lip measurements also generally correlate with a shift from masculine to more feminine anthropometric proportions. Lip lifts therefore have become a useful component of facial feminization, and are a powerful tool for changing the gender-associated appearance of the lower facial third. We have adopted a modified "bullhorn" technique to achieve a subtle lift while minimizing visible incisions.

The goals of the lip lift as a gender-confirming procedure are, foremost, to reduce the height of the cutaneous upper lip, increase the visible red vermilion, and enhance pout while attaining an appropriate amount of dental show and minimizing visible scarring. We herein describe the senior author's preferred technique for male-to-female lip lifts in the context of traditional lip rejuvenation procedures and with important considerations for transgender patients.

THE UPPER LIP
Anatomy

The upper lip should be considered with regards to its anatomic and aesthetic subunits. It is a trilaminar structure with the middle foundational layer consisting of the superior half of the sphincteric

Disclosures: None of the authors has a financial interest in any of the products, devices, or drugs mentioned in this article. No funding was received from any external sources.
Hansjörg Wyss Department of Plastic Surgery, New York University Langone Health, 305 East 33rd Street, New York, NY 10016, USA
* Corresponding author.
E-mail address: Rachel.Bluebond-Langner@nyumc.org

Facial Plast Surg Clin N Am 27 (2019) 261–266
https://doi.org/10.1016/j.fsc.2019.01.004
1064-7406/19/© 2019 Elsevier Inc. All rights reserved.

orbicularis oris with contributions from the buccinator and lip elevators. The orbicularis oris is juxtaposed by the mucosa posteriorly containing multiple minor salivary glands. The outermost layer of the lip is divided into the skin and the vermilion. The upper lip contains hair-bearing skin with numerous sweat and sebaceous glands underneath, which is a thick layer of subcutaneous fat. The red vermilion represents a transition from skin (at the white roll or vermilion border) to oral mucosa (at the wet-dry line) and consists of a thin layer of epithelium absent of glandular elements with a rich underlying capillary network. The philtrum, or philtral groove, is the central focal point of the upper lip, defined on each side by philtral columns formed from insertions of the contralateral orbicularis oris with contributions from the levator labii superioris inferiorly.

The aesthetic boundaries of the cutaneous upper lip include the vermilion border inferiorly, the nasal sill and alar bases superiorly, and the nasolabial fold and oral commissures laterally. The upper lip is further divided into aesthetic subunits including two medial subunits comprising the philtral groove and two lateral subunits each formed by a philtral column and lateral lip adjacent to the nasolabial fold.[10] For the purposes of lip lifts, relevant surface anatomy measurements include the subnasale to labiale superius (depth of cupid's bow) in the midline, or philtral distance, and labiale superius to stomion measurement, or labial distance.[11] These measurements correlate to the upper lip cutaneous skin height and vermilion height, respectively, in the midline.

Aesthetic Ideals

Lip lifts performed as gender-confirming procedures must take into account the aesthetic ideals of the upper lip. These ideals include an upper lip cutaneous skin height (philtral distance) to vermilion height (labial distance) ratio of less than three,[11] and a short philtrum with symmetric and prominent philtral columns.[12] Post lip rejuvenation lip lifts have an ideal philtrum to upper vermilion ratio of 2 to 2.9 and visible upper to lower vermilion of 0.75 to 0.8.[11,13] In general, a greater upper vermilion height, or vermilion show, has been found to be more attractive.[14] These ratios should be taken into consideration when planning gender-affirming lip lifts to ensure that results are not only more biologically "female," but also aesthetically pleasing.

The Male and Female Upper Lip

Differences in the appearance of the male and female upper lip are the basis of lip lifts as gender-affirming procedures for transgender females. Overall upper lip height, as measured from supramentale to stomion, is greater in males than females (average 23.6 vs 20.6 mm, respectively).[15] Subsequently, females tend to have a greater ideal upper incisor show in repose compared with males (around 4 vs 2 mm, respectively). The proportion of upper lip cutaneous skin height to upper vermilion height is also greater in males.[16] However, upper vermilion height itself is not different between males and females.[15,17] Along these lines, increased upper vermilion height has been found to be more attractive in males and females.[14]

PREOPERATIVE CONSIDERATIONS

All gender-affirming surgeries should follow the recommendations of the World Professional Association for Transgender Health Standards of Care. As with other gender-affirming procedures, the persistence of gender dysphoria, the patient's capacity to make fully informed decisions and consent to treatment, and the presence of any significant medical or mental health disorders should be assessed and documented.[18] Although a lip lift does not require referrals from mental health providers,[18] ongoing mental health support is an important aspect of comprehensive care during gender-affirming procedures. Aside from a general medical and surgical history, particular attention should be paid to prior facial feminization procedures, especially rhinoplasty or mentoplasty, and any history of orthognathic surgery.

Classification systems described for lip rejuvenation can provide a useful template for analysis.[11] Important factors to consider include philtral height, labial height (vermilion height), and dental show. The position of the oral commissures and lower lip vermilion height and fullness are also taken into consideration. Absolute measurements and relative proportions are important. Surrounding features should be evaluated including lower facial height, chin projection, nasal tip projection, nasolabial angle, and alar base width, at a minimum. An upper lip lift is roughly simulated with bimanual traction to estimate the appropriate amount of resection and gauge a general postoperative result.[3] Any preoperative asymmetry should also be noted and shown to the patient.

Underlying bony anatomy and general cephalometric concepts must be taken into account when planning soft tissue changes. Patients with vertical maxillary excess will have increased upper incisor show in repose and a "long face," whereas those with vertical maxillary deficiency will have an absence of incisal show on smiling. Occlusive patterns have a similar effect on upper lip height because a more protruded maxilla (sella-nasion-A point angle >82°) may convey the appearance of decreased upper lip height. Changes from manipulation of the soft tissues may therefore be exaggerated or minimized by the underlying bony and should be taken into account.

Proper patient selection and evaluation is critical in optimizing outcomes. Patients that will benefit from a lip lift have an increased philtral height without significant upper incisal show in repose. Patients with a wider alar base will have a more effective lateral lift as the excisions extend to the perialar creases, whereas those with a narrower base width may only achieve adequate central lift. A nasal base to lip-width ratio of 1:2 has been suggested to prevent inadequate lateral lifting.[19] Fair-skinned patients with no history of hypertrophic scarring or keloid formation and thinner skin, and older patients, tend to form less readily noticeable scars. Scarring history is particularly important in lip lifts because poor scarring is readily noticeable. It is critical to discuss the scar preoperatively, especially in young patients, and even draw it out for the patient.

Patient education through a process of shared decision-making is paramount in the preoperative work-up. Standard details on the procedure, recovery, and potential complications should be appropriately communicated and patient comprehension ensured. Important points include expected time to healing, duration of postoperative swelling, and evolution of scar appearance. This process additionally involves listening to the patient's own goals and mutually arriving at realistic expectations of postoperative results for this procedure. Preoperative and postoperative images from prior patients are helpful in this regard.

Although top surgery and genital surgery are routinely covered by insurance, facial feminization procedures are often categorized by insurance providers as "aesthetic." Although these operations are as effective in treating gender dysphoria in certain cases, patients must understand the financial implications of this labeling by insurance providers. Fees and patient costs should be discussed and agreed on preoperatively.

SURGICAL TECHNIQUE
Markings

Preoperative markings are performed with the patient in the sitting position before infiltration of local anesthetic. The superior incision line (final scar line) is marked at the junction of the nasal base and upper lip. This line proceeds from the alar base, along the inside of the nasal sill and across the base of the columella (**Fig. 1**). The superior line is similarly drawn on the contralateral side, ensuring symmetry. Vertical lines at the philtral columns and alar bases are then drawn as for reference. The planned amount of skin excision is measured with calipers at these points based on the desired amount of upper lip height and incisal show. This height is usually from 5 to 10 mm and is approximated with bimanual traction or pinch technique. The inferior incision line is then drawn to parallel the superior line, ensuring symmetry between the two sides unless corrections are necessary to correct baseline asymmetry. Markings are finally rechecked and remeasured with calipers.

Operative Steps

The procedure is performed either under local anesthesia with sedation or general anesthesia. The incision lines and planned resection are infiltrated with 1% lidocaine with 1:200,000 epinephrine and adequate time for vasoconstriction is allowed. The incisions are made sharply and dissection is carried to the orbicularis oris with electrocautery. The skin and subcutaneous tissue of the planned excision are then removed off of the muscle and hemostasis is obtained. Wound closure is achieved with 5–0 Vicryl suture in the deep dermal layer and interrupted 6–0 nylons for the epidermis. Meticulous technique during

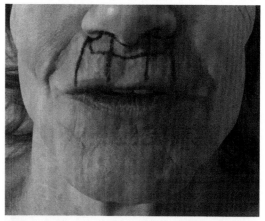

Fig. 1. Preoperative markings for gender-affirming lip lift. The planned scar line is outlined along the nasal base, running around the alar bases, nasal sill, and columella. Vertical lines are drawn along the philtral columns and at the lateral edges of the alar bases to ensure symmetry. The planned height of excision is estimated using bimanual traction on the upper lip and the lower incision line is measured based on the desired amount of upper incisal show and final upper lip height.

closure is needed to achieve precise dermal and epidermal approximation and minimize aberrant scarring (**Fig. 2**). The wound is dressed with antibiotic ointment.

Postoperative Care

Patients are instructed to apply antibiotic ointment to the incision line for the first postoperative week. Showering is allowed after 48 hours. Postoperative swelling is to be expected and discussed with patients preoperatively. Head elevation, cool compresses, and avoidance of strenuous activity for the first week postoperatively are encouraged to minimize postoperative edema. Nylon sutures are removed in the office in 5 to 7 days after which small adhesive tape strips are applied for further tissue support. Patients are instructed to avoid sun exposure to the scar line for 1 year postoperatively and use sunscreen over the incision when outside. Secondary scar treatments are used, such as scar creams and silicone sheets, and adjunctive treatments including dermabrasion and laser therapy are considered for dissatisfaction with scarring after 6 months.

DISCUSSION

The goals of gender-affirming lip lifts align well with those of lip rejuvenation. These include decreasing the height of the cutaneous upper lip, and increasing vermilion show and upper lip pout. In gender-affirming cases, focus is placed on shortening the upper lip length to within a range that is among aesthetically pleasing female "norms" because total upper lip height and the ratio of philtral to labial height (cutaneous to vermilion height) are greater in males. Importantly, soft tissue changes should aim to achieve an appropriate amount of upper incisal show and balance with the patient's lower facial aesthetics. As usual, undercorrection is better than overcorrection, and measured changes must be precise and tailored to the individual patient's facial profile. That said, a subtle amount of overcorrection accommodates for eventual upper lip descent over time postoperatively. An upper lip lift provides additional benefits of increase upper vermilion show and upper lip pout, which tend to be more aesthetically desirable in males and females.

A variety of different surgical techniques have been described to augment the lips and shorten the subnasal upper lip skin. The original bullhorn technique was described more than 40 years ago,[2] and has persisted as a common method of lip lifting. Several other types of indirect lip lifts have been designed to better address the philtrum[4,20] or lateral lip subunits,[21] conceal scars,[3] or minimize incisions.[22] The traditional subnasal bullhorn or seagull lip lift and its modifications are often used in feminization of the face.[1,23,24] We similarly use this technique because it allows varying degrees of lift with a concealed scar at the nasal base.

Certain differences between gender-affirming lip lifts and lip rejuvenation lifts should be recognized. Gender-affirming lifts primarily focus on shortening the nasal base-to-vermilion border

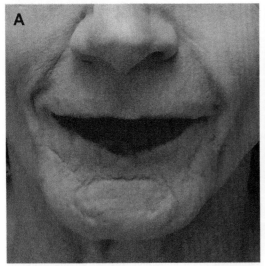
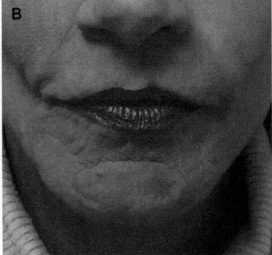

Fig. 2. (*A*) Preoperative photograph of a transgender female. Note the long philtral length (nasal sill to vermilion border height) and minimal vermilion show. (*B*) Postoperative photograph at 3 months showing decreased nasal base to vermilion border length and increased, symmetric vermilion height with scars along nasal base.

distance because this has been found to be the significant difference between male and female upper lip anthropometric proportions.[15,16] Although increased vermilion show and lip pout have been found to be aesthetically pleasing, these are of secondary importance in gender-affirming procedures because these traits are similar between males and females.[15,17] Furthermore, transgender females desiring a more feminine lower facial third may not have an increased philtral height amenable to lifting. Performing an excision in these patients may lead to undesirable dental show and "gummy" smile, which is difficult to correct. Overresection in any case can have a similar undesirable outcome. Certain authors have suggested that no more than 25% of the upper lip height from nasal sill to vermilion border should be excised in facial feminization cases.[23]

Patient selection and precise surgical technique are critical in minimizing complications. Scarring is usually the primary concern of the patients, and although is inevitable, is concealed with correct incision placement at the interface of the nasal and upper lip aesthetic subunits and with meticulous surgical technique, including gentle tissue handling and precise dermal apposition. Adverse scarring has been reported from 1% to 5% of indirect lip cases in patient series.[3,4] Secondary treatments including dermabrasion, silicone sheets, and laser therapy are used for visible scarring.[25] Older patients tend to heal with less noticeable scars and also have greater preoperative lip ptosis making them better candidates for lip lifts. Patient with darker complexion or history of wide/elevated scars should be counseled preoperatively.

Wound breakdown is uncommon, but is managed with local wound care and secondary scar revision as needed. Other complications include asymmetry, and overcorrection or undercorrection. Although undercorrection can be revised, overcorrection is difficult to treat, and therefore surgeons should err toward a subtler lift, particularly in patients with vertical maxillary excess or borderline incisor show. Alar base distortion is more common with endonasal techniques,[3] but can also be problematic with larger lifts or significant tension at the incision.

Satisfactory aesthetic outcomes similarly rely on selection of appropriate surgical candidates and meticulous preoperative planning. Both the surgeon and the patient must understand what the lip lift can and cannot achieve with regards to feminizing the perioral region. Subnasal lip lifts primarily address the central upper lip and are less effective laterally. This discrepancy is further exaggerated in patients with a narrow alar base width. Postoperatively, decreased lateral lift may manifest as downturned lateral commissures, which usually resolves after a few weeks. Variations in philtral morphology may also affect lip lift results. Central insertion of nonparallel philtral columns has been suggested to result in lateralization of the columns' insertion with lip lift and a more truncated lip appearance.[26] Furthermore, the nasal sill should be taken to consideration because patients with a more prominent sill can better hide incisional scars in the subsill crease.[27]

Lip lifts performed for lip rejuvenation are often combined with lip augmentation. Dermal grafts are performed simultaneously to increase vermilion border fullness.[23] Various lip fillers can also be used to enhance the vermilion and upper lip pout. Because gender-affirming lip lifts are primarily focused on shortening the subcutaneous subnasal lip, or philtral distance, adjunct lip augmentation is performed less frequently as a concomitant procedure. Providers, however, must still be cognizant of patients' history of prior lip fillers. These substances may include non–Food and Drug Administration–approved materials, such as injectable silicone, which can cause significant local inflammatory reactions, granulomas, and infection requiring excision.

Outcomes in facial feminization are continuing to be defined. Particularly with less-commonly performed procedures, such as lip lifts, there is a need for outcomes-based research. Patient-reported outcomes have been reported in facial feminization,[28] but overall, validated measures of these outcomes are lacking for gender-affirming procedures.[29] Moving forward, better assessment of short-term objectives and long-term patient satisfaction will help better define the aesthetic ideals for gender-affirming lip lifts and the optimal techniques to achieve these outcomes.

SUMMARY

Lip lifts are a powerful tool for facial feminization that allow for shortening of the height of the cutaneous upper lip skin to create a more feminine lower facial-third. Lip lifts also provide more aesthetically pleasing increased vermilion height and lip pout. Traditional subnasal bullhorn lifts work well for facial feminization in appropriately selected patients. There are several important characteristics to consider in evaluation of patients including skin type, soft tissue characteristics of the lip and nose, and underlying bone structure that can affect the efficacy of the lip. Proper patient selection, precise preoperative planning to avoid overcorrection and asymmetry, and meticulous surgical technique to minimize visible scarring optimize outcomes.

REFERENCES

1. Morrison SD, Vyas KS, Motakef S, et al. Facial feminization: systematic review of the literature. Plast Reconstr Surg 2016;137:1759–70.
2. Cardoso AD, Sperli AE. Rhitidoplasty of the upper lip. In: Hueston JT, editor. Transactions of the fifth international congress of plastic and reconstructive surgery. Melbourne (Australia): Butterworhts; 1971. p. 1127–9.
3. Raphael P, Harris R, Harris SW. The endonasal lip lift: personal technique. Aesthet Surg J 2014;34: 457–68.
4. Austin HW. The lip lift. Plast Reconstr Surg 1986;77: 990–4.
5. Li YK, Ritz M. The modified bull's horn upper lip lift. J Plast Reconstr Aesthet Surg 2018;71(8):1216–30.
6. Mommaerts MY, Blythe JN. Rejuvenation of the ageing upper lip and nose with suspension lifting. J Craniomaxillofac Surg 2016;44:1123–5.
7. Weston GW, Poindexter BD, Sigal RK, et al. Lifting lips: 28 years of experience using the direct excision approach to rejuvenating the aging mouth. Aesthet Surg J 2009;29:83–6.
8. Penna V, Iblher N, Bannasch H, et al. Proving the effectiveness of the lip lift for treatment of the aging lip: a morphometric evaluation. Plast Reconstr Surg 2010;126:83e–4e.
9. Lee DE, Hur SW, Lee JH, et al. Central lip lift as aesthetic and physiognomic plastic surgery: the effect on lower facial profile. Aesthet Surg J 2015;35: 698–707.
10. Burget GC, Menick FJ. Aesthetic restoration of one-half the upper lip. Plast Reconstr Surg 1986;78: 583–93.
11. Raphael P, Harris R, Harris SW. Analysis and classification of the upper lip aesthetic unit. Plast Reconstr Surg 2013;132:543–51.
12. Suryadevara AC. Update on perioral cosmetic enhancement. Curr Opin Otolaryngol Head Neck Surg 2008;16:347–51.
13. Perkins SW, Sandel HD. Anatomic considerations, analysis, and the aging process of the perioral region. Facial Plast Surg Clin North Am 2007;15: 403–7, v.
14. Penna V, Fricke A, Iblher N, et al. The attractive lip: a photomorphometric analysis. J Plast Reconstr Aesthet Surg 2015;68:920–9.
15. Anic-Milosevic S, Mestrovic S, Prlic A, et al. Proportions in the upper lip-lower lip-chin area of the lower face as determined by photogrammetric method. J Craniomaxillofac Surg 2010;38:90–5.
16. Farkas LG, Katic MJ, Hreczko TA, et al. Anthropometric proportions in the upper lip-lower lip-chin area of the lower face in young white adults. Am J Orthod 1984;86:52–60.
17. Fernandez-Riveiro P, Suarez-Quintanilla D, Smyth-Chamosa E, et al. Linear photogrammetric analysis of the soft tissue facial profile. Am J Orthod Dentofacial Orthop 2002;122:59–66.
18. The World Professional Association for Transgender Health. Standards of care for the health of transsexual, transgender, and gender nonconforming people. 7th version 2011. Available at: https://www.wpath.org/media/cms/Documents/Web Transfer/SOC/Standards of Care V7 - 2011 WPATH.pdf. Accessed April 10, 2018.
19. Waldman SR. The subnasal lift. Facial Plast Surg Clin North Am 2007;15:513–6, viii.
20. Gonzalez-Ulloa M. The aging upper lip. Ann Plast Surg 1979;2:299–303.
21. Marques A, Brenda E. Lifting of the upper lip using a single extensive incision. Br J Plast Surg 1994;47: 50–3.
22. Echo A, Momoh AO, Yuksel E. The no-scar lip-lift: upper lip suspension technique. Aesthetic Plast Surg 2011;35:617–23.
23. Altman K. Facial feminization surgery: current state of the art. Int J Oral Maxillofac Surg 2012;41:885–94.
24. Bellinga RJ, Capitan L, Simon D, et al. Technical and clinical considerations for facial feminization surgery with rhinoplasty and related procedures. JAMA Facial Plast Surg 2017;19:175–81.
25. Holden PK, Sufyan AS, Perkins SW. Long-term analysis of surgical correction of the senile upper lip. Arch Facial Plast Surg 2011;13:332–6.
26. Georgiou CA, Benatar M, Bardot J, et al. Morphologic variations of the philtrum and their effect in the upper lip lift. Plast Reconstr Surg 2014;134: 996e–7e.
27. Ponsky D, Guyuron B. Comprehensive surgical aesthetic enhancement and rejuvenation of the perioral region. Aesthet Surg J 2011;31:382–91.
28. Raffaini M, Magri AS, Agostini T. Full facial feminization surgery: patient satisfaction assessment based on 180 procedures involving 33 consecutive patients. Plast Reconstr Surg 2016;137: 438–48.
29. Andreasson M, Georgas K, Elander A, et al. Patient-reported outcome measures used in gender confirmation surgery: a systematic review. Plast Reconstr Surg 2018;141:1026–39.

Chondrolaryngoplasty— Thyroid Cartilage Reduction

Angela Sturm, MD[a,b], Scott R. Chaiet, MD, MBA[c,*]

KEYWORDS

- Tracheal shave • Adam's apple • Thyroid notch • Chondrolaryngoplasty • Transgender
- Transfeminine • Facial feminization surgery

KEY POINTS

- Chondrolaryngoplasty, or reduction in the thyroid cartilage, is the only treatment for an enlarged Adam's apple because the thyroid cartilage does not respond to gender-affirming hormonal therapy.
- Reconstructive procedures such as chondrolaryngoplasty are not optional in any meaningful sense but are understood to be medically necessary for the treatment of those with gender dysphoria.
- The chondrolaryngoplasty incision should be made cephalad to the thyroid cartilage in the cervicomental angle; a direct approach leaves a telltale neck scar, dangerously marking the patient's status, and it can scar to deeper structures, leading to a depressed scar that moves with swallowing or talking.
- Direct visualization with an endoscope combined with an external approach in reduction chondrolaryngoplasty can help to avoid damage to the vocal cord attachment as well as underreduction of the thyroid prominence.

INTRODUCTION

Pomus Adamus or Adam's apple, a prominent thyroid notch, is a result of the effect of testosterone on the thyroid cartilage of the larynx. Until puberty, the dimensions of the thyroid cartilage are similar in most larynges. After the increase in testosterone, the thyroid cartilage will grow larger and the superior aspect more prominent, both "masculine" physical characteristics. Many transfeminine patients find the Adam's apple distressing as an unwanted indication of that person's transgender status. In the facial feminization practice of Douglass Osterhout, MD, DDS, many sought their first surgical intervention for a prominent Adam's apple.[1] And in the 2015 US Transgender Survey, 4% of respondents with male on their original birth certificate had this procedure; however, 29% wanted the surgery 1 day while 29% were unsure.[2]

Chondrolaryngoplasty, or reduction in the thyroid cartilage, is the only treatment for those with gender dysphoria due to pomus Adamus because the thyroid cartilage does not respond to gender-affirming hormonal therapy such as soft tissue of the face. Pomus Adamus can not only be a large contributor to gender dysphoria but may also put that patient at risk for physical harm. In the 2015 US Transgender Survey, 48% of respondents experienced denial of equal treatment, verbal harassment, and/or were physically attacked

Disclosure Statement: The authors have nothing to disclose.
a Department of Otolaryngology–Head and Neck Surgery, University of Texas Medical Branch, 301 University Boulevard, Galveston, TX 77555-0521, USA; b Facial Plastic Surgery Associates, 6655 Travis Street, Suite 900, Houston, TX 77030, USA; c Division of Otolaryngology–Head and Neck Surgery, Department of Surgery, University of Wisconsin School of Medicine and Public Health, 600 Highland Avenue, CSC K4/7, Madison, WI 53792, USA
* Corresponding author.
E-mail address: chaiet@surgery.wisc.edu

Facial Plast Surg Clin N Am 27 (2019) 267–272
https://doi.org/10.1016/j.fsc.2019.01.005
1064-7406/19/© 2019 Elsevier Inc. All rights reserved.

because of being transgender. However, "those who said that others could usually or always tell that they were transgender (66%) were more likely to report having one or more of these experiences because of being transgender, in contrast to those who said that others could rarely or never tell that they were transgender (39%)."[2] So reducing the risk of being "outed" with surgery such as chondrolaryngoplasty effectively reduces harm in addition to treatment of gender dysphoria. In summary, chondrolaryngoplasty is an increasingly necessary operation in which surgeons should be competent.

EVALUATION

Chondrolaryngoplasty has been called various names throughout the literature including thyroid cartilage reduction, thyroid chondroplasty, laryngeal chondroplasty, and laryngochondroplasty. However, it is commonly called a tracheal shave; this is actually a misnomer and is a reduction of the thyroid cartilage rather than tracheal cartilage. Chondrolaryngoplasty is frequently requested by transfeminine patients but also anecdotally by cisgender men and even cisgender women. During the initial evaluation, patients may report the pomus Adamus causes gender dysphoria, a condition recognized in the Diagnostic and Statistical Manual of Mental Disorders, (DSM-5), published by the American Psychiatric Association. In its position statement for medical necessity for procedures such as chondrolaryngoplasty, the World Professional Association for Transgender Health states that the "medical procedures attendant to gender affirming/confirming surgeries are not "cosmetic" or "elective" or "for the mere convenience of the patient. These reconstructive procedures are not optional in any meaningful sense, but are understood to be medically necessary for the treatment of the diagnosed condition."[3]

Facial feminization surgery, an umbrella term that includes chondrolaryngoplasty, can significantly improve the quality of life for patients. In one review of patients who underwent facial feminization, all of the patients responded positively to a quality of life survey; when these patient outcomes were reviewed by 2 independent surgeons they were rated "very much improved" (87.8%) or "significantly improved" (12.1%).[4] Therefore, chondrolaryngoplasty should be viewed as medically necessary for gender dysphoria and can greatly improve quality of life.

ANATOMY

The thyroid cartilage is a shield-shaped structure composed of bilateral quadrilateral vertical laminae, which join together anteriorly forming a dihedral angle that is open posteriorly. The superior thyroid notch is formed by the fusion of the anterior borders of the 2 laminae. The anterior prominence of the thyroid cartilage is composed of the superior thyroid notch and the superior one-third of the laminae. Neck and pharyngeal muscles attach along the oblique line, lateral and posterior to the anterior prominence. Above the thyroid cartilage attaches the thyrohyoid membrane. The internal laryngeal nerve, a branch of the superior laryngeal nerve, penetrates the thyrohyoid membrane in its posterior half, cephalad to the superior laryngeal artery and vein and to the superior margin of the thyroid cartilage **Fig. 1**A. Care must be taken in this region as branches of this nerve supply sensation to the laryngeal structures above the glottis. The external branch of the superior laryngeal nerve descends along the posterior border of the thyroid cartilage, protected by the thyrohyoid muscle; the recurrent laryngeal nerve enters the larynx beneath the posteroinferior margin of the cricothyroid muscle.[5]

On the posterior thyroid cartilage lamina, the epiglottis inserts by means of the thyroepiglottic ligament well below the superior thyroid notch. Below this structure and protected by it are located the insertions of the false vocal cords and inferior to the false cords are the attachments

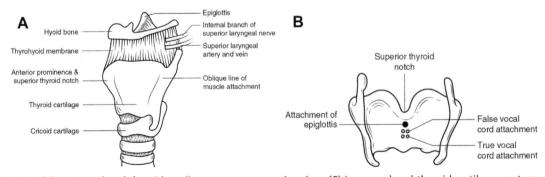

Fig. 1. (*A*) Laryngeal and thyroid cartilage anatomy, anterior view. (*B*) Laryngeal and thyroid cartilage anatomy, posterior view.

of the true vocal cords.[6] The attachment is referred to as the Broyle tendon.[6] The true vocal cords attach at the anterior commissure of the larynx to the posterior lamina of the thyroid cartilage approximately half way up the height of the cartilage according to topographic studies[6] (**Fig. 1**B). There is anatomic variation in the attachment that has also been described as between the superior one-third and interior two-thirds of the posterior aspect of the thyroid cartilage, which is why determining the exact location of each patient's true vocal cords is critical.[7]

At puberty, testosterone enlarges the larynx significantly, particularly the thyroid cartilage. The anteroposterior diameter of the larynx nearly doubles.[8] The effect of testosterone also causes the anterior angle of fusion of the 2 laminae to be more acute at 90°, whereas the "female" larynx or those without significant testosterone influence are wider and closer to 120°. The larger size of the superior thyroid notch and acute angle of laminae cause anterior projection that becomes more visible at rest and with talking and swallowing.

PROCEDURE

Chondrolaryngoplasty was described by Wolfort and Parry in 1975.[5] The optimal result involves removal of all anteriorly projecting thyroid cartilage while minimizing the risk of destabilizing the attachment of the epiglottis by the thyroepiglottic ligament, and anterior commissure tendon, which could cause permanent change to deepen the patient's voice, a particularly concerning complication for transfeminine patients who do not desire a deeper, more masculine voice[9] (**Fig. 2**).

Chondrolaryngoplasty can be performed alone or in combination with other procedures. If alone, this is often performed as an outpatient surgery under local anesthesia, intravenous sedation, or general anesthesia with either endotracheal intubation or laryngeal mask airway depending on patient and surgeon preference. When performed with other procedures, chondrolaryngoplasty is frequently the first procedure performed.[1,9]

The incision has been described directly over the thyroid cartilage; however, this leaves a telltale neck scar and can dangerously mark the patient's status. In addition, it can scar to deeper structures leading to a depressed scar that moves with swallowing or talking.[1] Therefore, it is recommended that the horizontal incision be made more cephalad in the cervicomental angle. Placement of the incision at this site reduces the chance of visibility and avoids the possibility of creating a retracted, mobile scar.[9] An anterior neck approach directly over the thyroid cartilage may be appropriate if other procedures are planned to modify the voice pitch[1,10] (**Fig. 3**).

After the skin incision is made, the subcutaneous plane is dissected. The anterior cervical vessels are identified and preserved if possible by lateral retraction; if necessary they are ligated and transected. The investing layer of the deep cervical fascia and then the middle cervical fascia are divided vertically.[5,11] The paired sternothyroid and thyrohyoid muscles are retracted laterally via a midline dissection plane. The superior one-third of the thyroid cartilage is exposed. The perichondrium is then incised along the superior rim of the thyroid laminae, with lateral dissection starting at a midpoint between the superior thyroid notch and oblique line proceeding to the thyroid notch medially[5] (**Fig. 4**A). A lateral dissection along the superior border can injure the superior laryngeal nerve, and care is also taken to stay on the rim with the incision to prevent entering the thyrohyoid membrane and preserve its attachment to the perichondrium of the posterior thyroid cartilage.[9,12]

A subperichondrial dissection is performed internally and externally using a Cottle elevator to reflect the perichondrium and expose the cartilage. The internal surface of the superior thyroid notch is elevated no farther inferiorly than the thyroepiglottic ligament; dissection beyond this point may destabilize the epiglottis and damage the vocal cord attachment. A curved hook can be

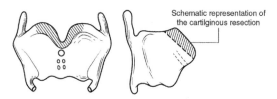

Fig. 2. Cartilage able to be excised in chondrolaryngoplasty surgery, with removal of all anteriorly projecting thyroid cartilage and preservation of the anterior commissure tendon.

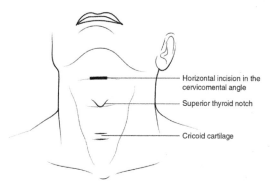

Fig. 3. Markings of skin incision, superior thyroid notch, and cricoid cartilage.

used on the posterior edge of the thyroid cartilage in the midline at the base of the notch to give superior-anterior retraction to perform anterior surface subperichondrial dissection.[9] Next, the superior thyroid notch, upper part of the laryngeal prominence, and prominent superior zone of the lateral laminae are excised by scalpel or rongeur. The surgeon should keep in mind that the procedure can become more challenging as people age and the cartilage ossifies requiring a saw or burrs. The internal structures are protected with an instrument such as a fine malleable retractor. The thyrohyoid membrane should be preserved because damage can place the superior laryngeal nerve in danger causing anesthesia of the larynx and possible aspiration[11] (**Fig. 4**B).

Removal of thyroid cartilage should be performed incrementally to achieve the appropriate contour. If using a rongeur, use extremely small bites to avoid fracturing the thyroid cartilage,

particularly if there is ossification.[1] However, the safety of placing small holes through the laryngeal cartilage has been established.[13] The edges can be smoothed with a burr to refine the contouring, if necessary. Then, the perichondrium is sutured over the resected cartilage with a 5-0 Vicryl suture (**Fig. 4**C). The fascia of the neck is reapproximated and the skin incision is closed in layers.[7] A small rubber catheter for drainage is optional.[5] The incision can be covered with a small adhesive dressing or a compression dressing overnight.

Conrad and Spiegel recommend a combined endoscopic and external approach to reduction chondrolaryngoplasty to avoid damage to the vocal cord attachment as well as underreduction of the thyroid prominence.[6,9] To perform the endoscopic-assisted chondrolaryngoplasty, general anesthesia is recommended. The incision and approach are identical to what is described earlier. Once the perichondrium of the thyroid

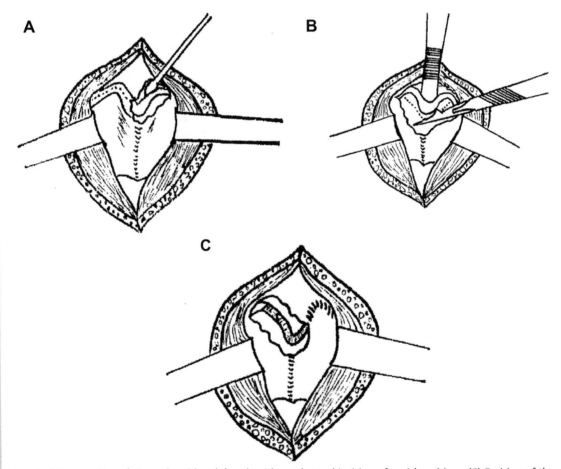

Fig. 4. (A) Retraction of sternothyroid and thyrohyoid muscles and incision of perichondrium. (B) Excision of the superior thyroid notch and anterior laryngeal prominence by scalpel and protection of internal structures. Excision may also be performed by rongeur, saw, or burrs. (C) The perichondrium is sutured over the resected cartilage followed by layered closure of fascia and skin. (*From* Giraldo F, de Grado J, Montes J. Aesthetic reductive thyroid chondroplasty. Int J Oral Maxillofac Surg 1997;26(1):21; with permission.)

cartilage is reflected, either a Keith needle or a 22 gauge needle is inserted through the cartilage into the laryngeal lumen a few millimeters above the midpoint of the anterior vertical height of the cartilage. Under direct visualization with an endoscope, the position of the needle in relation to the anterior commissure of the true vocal cords is verified (**Fig. 5**). At least 2 mm of cartilage above the superior surface of the true vocal cords should be left intact to provide support for the vocal cords and the thyroepiglottic ligament. Before removal, the external position of the marker needle is marked with a "V", with each limb in the vertical plane at a right angle to the anterior posterior line parallel to the vocal cords.

The patient can either be intubated with an endotracheal tube for the procedure and the needle is visualized with a laryngoscope[6] or the airway managed with a laryngeal mask airway (LMA) because the endotracheal tube can limit visualization of the anterior commissure and the needle.[9] If a laryngeal mask airway is used, a flexible laryngoscope is passed through the LMA for visualization. When combining chondrolaryngoplasty with other procedures, the LMA can be changed out for an endotracheal tube after the conclusion of the visualization portion of the chondrolaryngoplasty. The integrity of the vocal cords can be verified with a flexible laryngoscope at the conclusion of the cartilage excision or direct laryngoscopy at extubation.

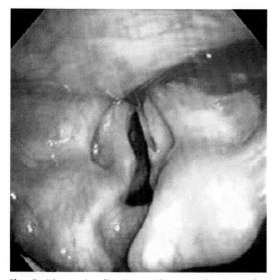

Fig. 5. Direct visualization with an endoscope of a needle inserted through the thyroid cartilage into the laryngeal lumen at least 2 mm above the superior surface of the true vocal folds. (*From* Spiegel JH, Rodriguez G. Chondrolaryngoplasty under general anesthesia using a flexible fiberoptic laryngoscope and laryngeal mask airway. Arch Otolaryngol Head Neck Surg 2008;134(7):704–8; with permission.)

MANAGING EXPECTATIONS

Overall patients are pleased with the outcome—up to 86% patient satisfaction rate.[10] If there is anteriorly projecting cartilage inferior to the level of the anterior commissure, a partial thickness shave may be possible in some situations; this does place the vocal cords at risk and leaving some thyroid cartilage in place is preferred.

Some patients have a large larynx and prominent superior thyroid notch. Because the larynx cannot be displaced posteriorly, these patients will likely have residual prominence of the larynx even after improving the contour of the thyroid cartilage. Because they will have a more feminine appearance but not ideal, the surgeon could proceed with appropriate patient expectations.[1] Mild edema of the cords is expected.[12] Also, the patient may have soft tissue edema for 3 to 6 months in the perioperative site camouflaging the final result, so should be counseled as such.[6]

MANAGEMENT OF COMPLICATIONS

Complications of chondrolaryngoplasty are rare. Conrad followed 10 patients for up to 2 years without complications.[6] Wolfort and colleagues[12] followed 31 patients up to 17 years and found the complications to be rare and usually transient with the most common being mild voice weakness; no patients experienced anesthesia of the larynx, neuralgia, or dysphagia. An anterior approach may lead to a wide, visible, retracted, or mobile neck scar that is extremely visible and can "out" the patient. Unsightly scars can be revised by excision and scar revision under local anesthesia. After excision of the scar, the layered closure is performed with either fat transfer or acellular dermis (eg, AlloDerm) is placed between the dermis and cervical fascia to prevent reformation of the scar tissue.[1] The appearance of the scar can also be improved with laser resurfacing.

Some patients may experience temporary narrowing of the vocal ranges and a sore throat that resolves in 3 to 4 days. Rarely, a patient may experience hoarseness that can last up to 6 months; Osterhout reported temporary lowering of the voice in 35% of his patients. This has historically been temporary. In the extremely rare occasion of disruption of the vocal cords, the change in voice could be permanent. Dysphagia could occur with disruption of the insertion of the epiglottis, although this has not been reported in the literature.

Endoscopic verification of the position of the vocal cords via a laryngeal mask airway provides excellent visualization of the anterior commissure of the vocal cords. However, this does require exchange for a more definitive airway for a longer case and could lead to anesthetic complications or at least a risk. Furthermore, the thyroid cartilage excision could lead to blood in the airway causing vocal cord irritation, which in light anesthesia can lead to laryngospasm without a definitive airway mediated by superior laryngeal nerve stimulation.[14] Laryngospasm occurred once in the series by Spiegel. However, rescue treatment of propofol, a low dosage of depolarizing agent, or increasing the depth of anesthesia can be performed. Topical lidocaine on the vocal cords at the time of endoscopy can also help reduce this risk.[9]

SUMMARY

Chondrolaryngoplasty is a medically necessary procedure that can greatly affect quality of life, particularly in transfeminine patients. Complications are rare and knowledge of the laryngeal anatomy can make them even less common. Outcomes are generally good and patient satisfaction is high, particularly with proper patient selection and management of expectations.

REFERENCES

1. Ousterhout DK. Facial feminization surgery: a guide for the transgendered woman. Omaha (NE): Addicus Books; 2010.
2. James SE, Herman JL, Rankin S, et al. The report of the 2015 U.S. transgender survey. Washington, DC: National Center for Transgender Equality; 2016.
3. World Professional Association for Transgender Health. Position statement on medical necessity of treatment, sex reassignment, and insurance coverage in the U.S.A. 2016. Available at: https://www.wpath.org/newsroom/medical-necessity-statement. Accessed June 17, 2018.
4. Raffaini M, Magri AS, Agostini T. Full facial feminization surgery: patient satisfaction assessment based on 180 procedures involving 33 consecutive patients. Plast Reconstr Surg 2016;137(2):438–48.
5. Wolfort FG, Parry RG. Laryngeal chondroplasty for appearance. Plast Reconstr Surg 1975;56(4):371–4.
6. Conrad K, Yoskovitch A. Endoscopically facilitated reduction laryngochondroplasty. Arch Facial Plast Surg 2003;5(4):345–8.
7. Giraldo F, de Grado J, Montes J. Aesthetic reductive thyroid chondroplasty. Int J Oral Maxillofac Surg 1997;26(1):20–2.
8. Gray H, Warwick R, Williams PL. Gray's anatomy. Edinburgh: Churchill Livingstone; 1980. p. 1229–36.
9. Spiegel JH, Rodriguez G. Chondrolaryngoplasty under general anesthesia using a flexible fiberoptic laryngoscope and laryngeal mask airway. Arch Otolaryngol Head Neck Surg 2008;134(7):704–8.
10. Matai V, Cheesman AD, Clarke PM. Cricothyroid approximation and thyroid chondroplasty: a patient survey. Otolaryngol Head Neck Surg 2003;128(6):841–7.
11. Al-Jassim AHH, Lesser THJ. Reduction of Adam's apple for appearance. Indian J Otolaryngol Head Neck Surg 2006;58(2):172–3.
12. Wolfort FG, Dejerine ES, Ramos DJ, et al. Chondrolaryngoplasty for appearance. Plast Reconstr Surg 1990;86(3):464–9.
13. O'Leary MA, Grillone GA. Injection laryngoplasty. Otolaryngol Clin North Am 2006;39(1):43–54.
14. Suzuki M, Sasaki CT. Laryngeal spasm: a neurophysiologic redefinition. Ann Otol Rhinol Laryngol 1977;86(2):150–7.

Moving?

Make sure your subscription moves with you!

To notify us of your new address, find your **Clinics Account Number** (located on your mailing label above your name), and contact customer service at:

Email: journalscustomerservice-usa@elsevier.com

800-654-2452 (subscribers in the U.S. & Canada)
314-447-8871 (subscribers outside of the U.S. & Canada)

Fax number: 314-447-8029

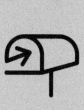

Elsevier Health Sciences Division
Subscription Customer Service
3251 Riverport Lane
Maryland Heights, MO 63043

*To ensure uninterrupted delivery of your subscription, please notify us at least 4 weeks in advance of move.

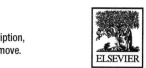

Printed and bound by CPI Group (UK) Ltd, Croydon, CR0 4YY

08/05/2025

01864741-0006